Hope and Destiny

HOPE AND DESTINY

The Patient's and Parent's Guide to Sickle Cell Disease and Sickle Cell Trait

ALLAN F. PLATT, JR., P.A.-C
AND
ALAN SACERDOTE, M.D.

Hilton Publishing Company • Roscoe, Illinois

Dedication

In memory of Ingrid Whittaker-Ware, Esq., who lived and shared her hopes and fulfilled her destiny.

Hilton Publishing Company
PO Box 737, Roscoe, IL 61073
815-885-1070
www.hiltonpub.com

Publisher's Cataloging-in-Publication
(Provided by Quality Books, Inc.)

Platt, Allan
    Hope & destiny; the patient's and parent's guide to sickle cell disease and sickle cell trait / by Allan Platt and Alan Sacerdote — 1st edition
    p. cm.
    Includes bibliographical references and index
    ISBN: 0–9675258–4–5

    1. Sickle cell anemia — Popular works
I. Sacerdote, Alan. II. Title

RC641.7.S5P53 2002   616.1'527
                                      QB102–200331

Printed and bound in the United States of America

CONTRIBUTORS

Dr. Benjamin Barrah. Private practice, Brooklyn, New York.

Melissa Creary. Research Associate and Sickle Cell Patient, Atlanta, Georgia

Heidy Dodard. College Student and Sickle Cell Patient, Atlanta, Georgia

Berrutha Harper. President Sickle Cell Parent Patient Group

Dr. Gregorio Hidalgo. Attending physician in hematology-oncology at Woodhull Medical and Mental Health Center, Brooklyn, New York.

Dr. Eko-Isenalumhe Arnold Imhona. Practices emergency medicine at Bronx-Lebanon Hospital, Bronx, New York.

P.A. Mark L'Eplattenier. Clinical coordinator and adjunct at S.U.N.Y. Health Science Center at Brooklyn Physician Assistant Program.

Sharon Lewin. Pre-med student at Brandeis University.

Dr. Beatrice Eleje Ony eador. Resident in internal medicine at Woodhull Medical and Mental Health Center, Brooklyn, New York.

Dr. Ehi Philip Osehobo. Practices internal medicine in East Point and Fayetteville, Georgia

Susan S. Platt, M.D. Internal Medicine Provider, Meridian Medical Group

Michelle Rodriguez. Patient Brooklyn, New York; scholarship student at Fashion Institute of Technology in Manhattan.

Nancy Sacerdote. B. A., Brooklyn College, M. A., Boston University.

Ingrid Whittaker-Ware, Esq. Patient Representative and lawyer

5/05

CONTRIBUTORS FROM THE GEORGIA COMPREHENSIVE SICKLE CELL CENTER AT GRADY HEALTH CENTER, ATLANTA, GEORGIA

JoAnn Beasley, R.N. Clinical Manager, Newborn Screening Coordinator the Georgia Comprehensive Sickle Cell Center at Grady Health System

Marietta Collins, Ph.D. Pediatric Psychologist at the Georgia Comprehensive Sickle Cell Center at Grady Health System

Melanie Jacob, M,D. M.P.H. Assistant Professor of Hematology/ Oncology, Winship Cancer Institute, Emory University School of Medicine, Attending Physician at the Georgia Comprehensive Sickle Cell Center at Grady Health System

James R. Eckman, M.D. Professor and Chief of Hematology/ Oncology, Winship Cancer Institute, Adjunct Professor of Pediatrics, Division of Medical Genetics Emory University School of Medicine, Medical Director, The Georgia Comprehensive Sickle Cell Center at Grady Health System

Beatrice Gee, M.D. Assistant Professor of Pediatric Hematology Oncology Morehouse School of Medicine, Attending Physician at the Georgia Comprehensive Sickle Cell Center at Grady Health System

Lewis Hsu, MD, Ph.D. Assistant Professor of Pediatrics, Division of Pediatric Hematology-Oncology Bone Marrow Transplant, Attending Physician at the Georgia Comprehensive Sickle Cell Center at Grady Health System

Patricia Myler. Multimedia Teacher and director—the Georgia Comprehensive Sickle Cell Center at Grady Health System

Artwork by Donna Dent, Research Assistant, The Georgia Comprehensive Sickle Cell Center and Emory University School of Medicine

CONTENTS

LIST OF TABLES

INTRODUCTION

Leviticus 17:14 . . . because the life of every creature is its blood.

Sickle cell disease is an inherited, lifelong problem that is located within the red blood cells of your body. A single chemical substitution in the protein hemoglobin, inside the red cell, causes that cell to take on a hard sickle shape instead of the normal soft, stretchable, doughnut shape that allows red cells to move through your blood vessels. The sickle shape causes blood flow blockages. It also causes the red blood cell to break apart (*hemolysis*), and this causes *anemia*, or a low red blood cell count. The body pains and other complications that people with sickle cell disease have are all caused by these blockages and by anemia.

In the United States, over 70,000 people have sickle cell disease. It is the most common genetic disease in this country. (It is also a serious global problem.) Each year about 1,000 babies are born in America with sickle cell disease. It is estimated that 3.5 million Americans carry the sickle cell trait—that is, they are carriers of one sickle cell gene, though they don't have the disease themselves. That is why African Americans, who are most likely to get the disease, need to be tested for sickle cell trait. Two people carrying the trait, neither of whom suffers any symptoms, may bring into the world a child with sickle cell disease who does suffer its serious effects.

Today, however, there's much good news. Now people with sickle cell disease live longer and more productive lives, thanks to early detection, preventive medications, better education about the disease, and new treatments for it.

Many new advances have occurred in the last fifteen years to prolong life and even to cure the disease:

- People with sickle cell disease now have a life expectancy at least into their mid 40s and 50s, due especially to new methods for preventing infections, strokes, and organ damage.
- Early detection of sickle cell through newborn screening, as well as preventive treatment, education and therapy, improves the chances of survival from infections and spleen problems from birth to age six.
- The first effective preventive medication (hydroxyurea) recently was approved by the Food and Drug Administration. This medication has reduced by half the number of pain episodes, the need for hospitalization, and the need for transfusion. New data suggest that it prolongs life.
- Bone-marrow transplants now can cure some sickle cell children who have a brother or sister to serve as a matched donor—though only the most serious cases merit the risk of going through this procedure.
- Screening children to find those at high risk of stroke allows effective preventive treatment to stop a stroke from happening.

Despite all of this good news, more needs to be done to educate patients and health care providers about sickle cell disease. Even though it is the most common genetic disease in the United States, research funding for it at all levels is very low because the number of patients is small and, often, the patient's economic status is low as well.

Still, much can be accomplished by motivated people working together for a common goal. The resources in this book can empower you, the reader, to become an informed, active member of the sickle cell community and to change lives for the better.

Because sickle cell disease is genetic, because it involves blood chemistry, and because it can strike many of the body's organs, it is harder to understand than diseases that strike single parts of the body.

This book explains clearly what you need to know about sickle cell disease and trait. It is based on the many questions parents, patients and friends have asked the staff of the Georgia Comprehensive Sickle Cell Center at Grady Memorial Hospital in Atlanta, Georgia, over a period of more than fifteen years.

PATIENTS' STORIES

We have included stories written by people with sickle cell disease to describe how the disease affects different age groups. From these stories and the stories posted on the Sickle Cell Information Center website, you will get encouragement, instruction, and hope. You may also want to tell your own story on the website, http://www.emory.edu/PEDS/SICKLE/ or on www.SCInfo.org. The people who tell these stories—parents and people with the disease who have learned to cope with it day by day—are the true heroes of this book.

A NOTE TO THE READER

Some readers may want to start this book at chapter three. The two opening chapters on how the blood works and how genetics works are sometimes technical. You may want to use the book by addressing your questions to it. That means, with the help of the table of contents and index, decide which subjects you want to start with, and get the answers from the book. After you've explored the book in that way, you may feel better prepared to take on the more technical questions.

PART ONE

THE ABCs OF SICKLE CELL DISEASE

CHAPTER 1

Understanding the Blood

Over five liters of blood constantly circulate through the tunnels called arteries, away from the lungs, and through the veins back to the lungs. Blood supplies food, oxygen, and messages to your body's organs and removes wastes, carbon dioxide, and old cell parts for recycling. Blood also helps the body heat and cool itself. It is truly the river of life.

PLASMA

Blood is made up of a fluid called plasma and three types of cells. Plasma contains the water, sugar, salt, hormones, proteins, and minerals necessary to keep cells alive. It is the fluid that carries the cells around the body to where they are needed. Plasma is filtered by the kidney where urine is made, the liver where protein is made and stored, and the spleen, where germs and old cells are removed.

WHITE CELLS

White blood cells are the defenders of the body. They help capture and fight invading germs and protect the body against foreign cancer cells, viruses, and chemicals. There are different types of white blood cells, each with a different mission and defense loca-

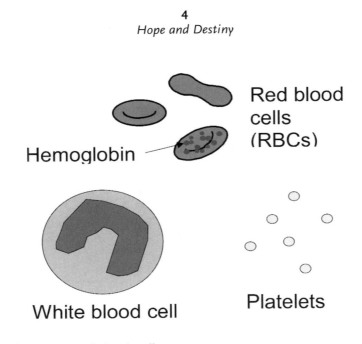

Red blood cells (RBCs)

Hemoglobin

White blood cell

Platelets

The Three Types of Blood Cells

tion. One type of white cell makes immune protein that fights bacteria, viruses and foreign proteins that enter the body. This immune reaction can be a bad thing when blood, bone marrow or another body part is transplanted or transfused as a treatment and the body attacks it. A rising white blood cell count may be the first sign of an infection attacking the body.

The white blood cells in people with sickle cell disease do not attack germs as well they do in people without sickle cell. The result can be increased infections.

PLATELETS

Platelets are the body's hole plugger-uppers. When the skin and blood vessels are cut or a hole is made, bleeding occurs. The platelets spring into action and cause the blood to form a jelly-like plug, called a *clot*, to block the hole and stop the bleeding. If there are not enough platelets around, you may not stop bleeding. If too many platelets are around, the blood may clot inside blood vessels where there is no hole. This can damage tissue because the blood flow to that area stops.

In people with sickle cell disease, the platelets are more active than in people without it. This increased activity can lead to increased clotting inside blood vessels where there is no hole.

RED CELLS

Red blood cells are the soft doughnut shaped (the raised fluffy kind) taxicabs that carry the oxygen you breathe to all your living cells, pick up the waste product, carbon dioxide, and carry it back to the lungs for you to breathe out. There are 25 trillion red blood cells in the body at any given instant. They are too small to be seen without the help of a microscope. (For example, there would be about fifty red blood cells in the space of a period at the end of this sentence.) The red cell's shape is perfectly designed to travel the narrow capillaries out in the far parts of the body (a capillary is a tiny blood vessel that connects larger blood vessels).

Red cells normally last 120 days. Then the covering, or membrane, breaks apart and the chemicals that make up the cells are recycled.

The red cell is the main actor in the drama of sickle cell disease. One small change in the chemical hemoglobin inside the red cell can change its shape and cause all of the problems we will talk about.

HEMOGLOBIN

The protein inside the red blood cell that does all of the work is called *hemoglobin*. It holds the oxygen that is picked up in the lungs, releases it out into the distant tissue, and holds the carbon dioxide for a trip back to the lungs for disposal. It is the hemoglobin that makes the red blood cells red, and gives blood its red color.

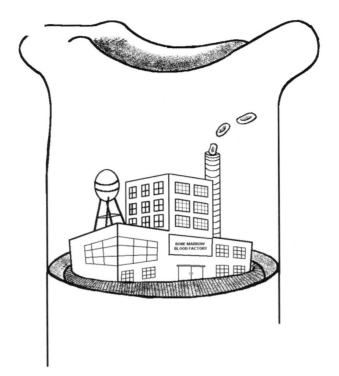

Hemoglobin with oxygen is "bright red" and hemoglobin that has given up its oxygen is "dark blue-red."

The way hemoglobin is made is determined by the DNA blueprint that every child inherits from each parent. There are normally three types of hemoglobin in each red blood cell: A, A2, and F or Fetal. Fetal hemoglobin is the main type babies have inside the womb. It tightly holds oxygen because the baby is not breathing inside the womb, and all oxygen comes from the mother across the placenta.

Once the baby is born, fetal hemoglobin is replaced by hemoglobin made according to the genetic blueprint. Normal hemoglobin (hemoglobin A) is made up of two types of protein chains: two alpha chains and two beta chains. Trouble starts when one amino acid called *glutamic acid* on the beta chain is substituted for another called *valine*.

BONE MARROW

The red cells, white cells and platelets are all made in the bone marrow, inside the big bones of the body. This is where stem cells make the cells needed for the blood according to the DNA blueprint inherited from each parent.

Anything that harms or stops the bone marrow factory can cause the red cell, white cell, and platelet number to fall and the person to become very ill.

The only cure available now for sickle cell disease is to kill a person's bone marrow with medications and replace it, or implant it, with marrow from a brother or sister. This changes the DNA blueprint to that of the donor.

BLOOD VESSELS

Blood is carried through the miles of tubing in the body called blood vessels. Arteries carry blood full of new oxygen from the lungs through the main pump, the heart, and out to smaller arterioles and even smaller capillaries. Arteries have muscles in their walls that can make the opening smaller, or if they relax can make the opening wider. Some capillaries are smaller than the diameter of the red cell, and the red cell must stretch to go through and deliver its life-giving oxygen. If the red cell becomes hard, or rigid, for any reason it can block blood flow through the capillary.

Once the blood flows through the capillaries and delivers its oxygen, it enters tubing called the *venule*, and then the larger vein for its trip back to the lungs for more oxygen. It is in the slow flowing venules where scientists suspect most of the sickling of the red cells occurs.

Sickle red cells are also stickier than non-sickle red cells and can become stuck to the blood vessel walls.

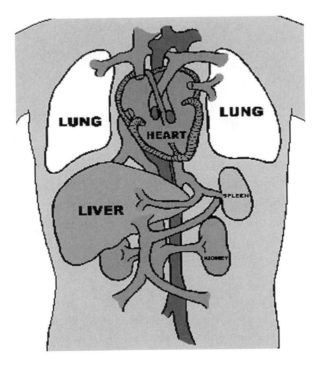

THE RED CELL CYCLE

Food containing iron, protein, B vitamins, folate—the building blocks for red blood cells and hemoglobin—is absorbed from the intestines. Nutrients are carried to the bone marrow factory in the middle of your large bones in the arms, legs, back, and hips. Here, red cells, white cells, and platelets are made. Infant red cells, called *reticulocytes*, are released into the blood stream and mature over two days. The red cell then is pumped around the body from the lungs to the tissues by the heart.

After its normal 120 day life, the red cell becomes easily damaged and breaks apart. The hemoglobin is released, and is broken down into a chemical called *bilirubin*. The iron and protein from the broken red cell are recycled and reused. Not eating the proper foods or any bleeding, like menstrual bleeding, can cause low iron, which can make you tired.

The kidney also helps keeps red cell production going. Inside the kidney are cells that sense the level of oxygen in the red cells. If the oxygen level is low, these cells in the kidney secrete a hormone, called *erythropoeitin*, that travels in the blood stream to the bone marrow and stimulates more red blood cell production. It is like a call from a retail store to a factory to order more product because the shelves are empty. If the kidneys become damaged, the erythropoietin level may fall and the bone marrow may slow down red blood cell production. This process can now be fixed with injections of manufactured erythropoietin (Epogen™ or Procrit™). If doctors need to increase red blood cell production for any reason, they can boost it by giving an injection of this hormone.

CAUSES OF ANEMIA

Anemia is a lower than normal number of red blood cells. You can get anemia by not eating foods rich in iron or getting enough vitamins, proteins, and fats to build the red cells in the bone marrow factory. The most common cause of anemia in the United States is lack of iron.

As you know, the bone marrow factory can be attacked by infections, drugs, or chemicals causing it to slow down production. Red blood cells can break apart before 120 days, weakening the system. This is called *hemolysis*. In sickle cell disease the red blood cells break apart in about fourteen days instead of the normal 120 days. This is the main cause of the low red blood cell counts. Bleeding can also cause anemia until the body replaces the lost cells. Anemia should be evaluated by your doctor to determine the cause.

CHAPTER 2

Understanding Genetics

GENETICS AND BLOOD DISEASE

Genetics is the science that deals with heredity—that determines or reads the blueprint for every organ, bone, body part, and cell of your body. Your blueprint is like a blueprint for a building. If a builder's blueprint is wrong, it might tell the builder to put a door where a water pipe should go. If the blueprint doesn't have enough girders to hold up the building, it could collapse.

Each cell in the human body has a genetic code blueprint that tells that cell what to make and what to do. This blueprint, or code, is passed from parents to child in the DNA in forty-six chromosomes—twenty-three from each parent. Your DNA blueprint determines your eye, hair, and skin color. It also determines the makeup of the hemoglobin inside your red blood cells.

HEMOGLOBINOPATHIES

A *mutation* or change in the DNA code blueprint can cause genetic diseases.

Hemoglobinopathies are a group of genetic diseases that occur because of a mutation that directs how hemoglobin is made. Because hemoglobin carries oxygen to all the parts of the body, the health of the hemoglobin determines the health of the body. If your hemoglobin is healthy, you'll be stronger and healthier.

The structure of the hemoglobin molecule can vary widely, but variations of only 1 percent can cause serious diseases such as sickle cell disease and other diseases called *thalassemias*. Thalassemia is an inherited hemoglobin problem where not enough of the alpha or beta chains that make up the hemoglobin structure are produced. Thus, you and I can carry a hemoglobin gene abnormality and not know about it because it does not show itself as disease.

HEMOGLOBIN S AND SICKLE CELL DISEASE—SS

We believe that the sickle cell mutation allowed human beings who lived in West Africa, where it first occurred, to better survive the threat that their gene pool might be destroyed by malaria, a red blood cell parasite. Those with sickle cell trait (one of many hemoglobin abnormalities that does not show itself as disease) still get malaria, but they have a better chance to survive it than those without the trait. Unfortunately, the existence of the trait made the disease possible. By mating, two persons with sickle cell trait may produce offspring with sickle cell disease.

It is important to tell your health care providers if you have sickle cell trait. It is also important for you to understand the symptoms that can show up under extreme conditions and to know how to avoid complications.

If you have sickle cell trait,

- You may pass this gene on to your children.
- You can be sure it will never turn into sickle cell disease.
- You can have a normal life without symptoms if you avoid extremes of dehydration, low oxygen, pressure changes, or extreme exhaustion.
- Certain occupations and recreational activities may cause problems.

• Travel to high altitudes or deep sea diving can bring on symptoms.

HEMOGLOBIN C AND SICKLE CELL DISEASE—SC

Sickle cell trait can form different combinations with other abnormal hemoglobins. In the one called Sickle C (SC), hemoglobin C combines with sickle cell trait. This combined version of two abnormal hemoglobins results in sickle cell disease—SC, much like sickle cell disease—SS, but milder in many respects.

Another possible combination, CC disease, causes a mild anemia, occasional joint and abdominal pain, enlarged spleen, and gallstones.

HEMOGLOBIN E AND SICKLE CELL DISEASE—SE

Still another hemoglobinopathy, called hemoglobin E disease, has become common in the United States because of the large number of immigrants from southeast Asia, where the disease originated. In this disease there is decreased production of hemoglobin and therefore smaller red blood cells.

While this disease causes a mild anemia and few other problems, its can be devastating. When hemoglobin E trait combines with a hemoglobin problem called *thalassemia,* a most serious disease, which we discuss next, results. Hemoglobin E and S may combine to form sickle cell disease—SE. This is rare and is reported to be a milder form of sickle cell disease.

THALASSEMIAS AND SICKLE CELL DISEASE—S BETA THALASSEMIA

The thalassemias are a group of diseases that make the body less able—or even *unable*—to use, or synthesize, one or more proteins *(globins)* that make up hemoglobin. A person who suffers from thalassemic disorder has less hemoglobin than normal available to make blood. The result can be anemia or other disorders.

ALPHA THALASSEMIAS

Thalassemias are described as *alpha* or *beta*. Alpha thalassemia affects the alpha chain of hemoglobin and beta thalassemia affects the beta chain of hemoglobin. While the alpha thalassemias are found primarily in people from China and southeast Asia, they are also seen sometimes in Black people. Immigration has made these diseases more common in the United States.

There is a wide range of alpha thalassemias found, depending on how many of the four alpha chains in a single hemoglobin molecule get produced. When only one chain of the four is missing, the person affected is normal and won't experience (nor will the doctor detect) any signs of the disease.

At the other extreme, babies conceived with all four alpha chains (or *copies*) missing die in the womb; they never get a chance to be born.

Two missing alpha chains means "thalassemia minor;" the person has thalassemia trait but will live a normal life.

If there are three missing chains, a set of diseases called "hemoglobin H diseases" will develop. Hemoglobin H diseases are a serious problem, because the severe breakdown of the red blood cells causes chronic anemia and a big spleen.

BETA THALASSEMIA

Beta thalassemias result from a mutation and occur in the beta chain manufacturing process. The mild form of beta thalassemia is called *beta thalassemia minor* because the anemia it causes is mild. Beta thalassemia does not require transfusion or other treatment.

People with this condition can live comfortably, but it is important that they be identified. Treating their anemia with iron, as a different kind of anemia would be treated, leads to iron overload and the deposit of iron into the body tissues.

In the severe form of beta thalassemia, termed *beta thalassemia major,* there is little or no production of beta chains, and the hemoglobin molecule is very unstable. Individuals with this disease need frequent blood transfusions in order to stay alive.

Thalassemia trait can combine with sickle cell trait to produce sickle cell disease S-beta thalassemia. This can be mild to very severe, like sickle cell disease — SS.

Another combination that can occur is between hemoglobin D and sickle cell trait. The clinical result is called SD disease. It resembles sickle cell disease but is less severe.

INCIDENCE OF SICKLE HEMOGLOBIN

In the Black population in the United States,

- the incidence of sickle cell trait is about 8 percent
- the incidence of hemoglobin C trait is about 3 percent
- the incidence of beta thalassemia trait is about 1.5 percent.

CHAPTER 3

Genetic Counseling

Proverbs 24:3 By wisdom a house is built, and through understanding it is established;

THE AIMS OF GENETIC COUNSELING

There is no cure for sickle cell anemia today except bone marrow transplants. But a couple who wish to have children can know in advance whether their child will carry the sickle cell trait and/or actually have sickle cell disease. With that knowledge, they can face the hard question of whether or not to bring into the world a child likely to suffer with sickle cell disease.

WHAT A GENETIC COUNSELOR DOES

A genetic counselor first

- learns the medical history of both parents
- orders blood tests
- orders chromosome analyses

Based on this information the counselor can then determine the chances that the parents will pass on a defective gene to their offspring.

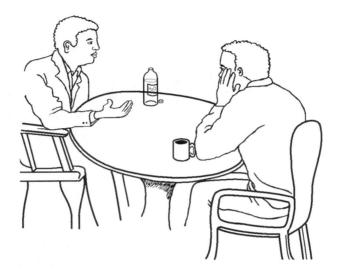

Besides informing prospective parents whether they are likely to pass on the defective gene, *the genetic counselor helps after the baby is born by ordering "screening" tests that allow precise diagnosis.* In many states such screening is mandatory. Screening tests make possible more effective treatment, and also let parents know what symptoms they may expect in their child.

If there is a chance that the couple will pass the sickle trait or disease to a baby, the counselor will talk to the parents about the resources they will need to raise a child with sickle cell disease. The counselor will also describe the effect the disease is likely to have on the parents' lives as well as the child's.

FINDING AND WORKING WITH A GENETIC COUNSELOR

You can find a genetic counselor by contacting your local health department as well as state genetic services coordinators. University hospitals are usually good sources of information because they are affiliated with medical schools and usually provide high quality medical care and research.

Table 1

Here is an outline of what the screening tests may tell the counselor and the parents

Case #	Parent #1	Parent #2	Children
1	Sickle cell disease Hb SS	Sickle cell disease Hb SS	100% of children -> sickle cell disease Hb SS
2	Sickle cell disease Hb SS	Sickle cell trait Hb AS	50% -> sickle cell trait Hb AS 50% -> sickle cell disease Hb SS
3	Sickle Cell Disease type SC or Hb SC	Normal Hb AA	50 % Trait Hb AS 50 % Trait Hb AC
4	Normal Hb AA	Normal Hb AA	100% normal Hb AA
5	Sickle Cell Trait Hb AS	Sickle Cell Trait Hb AS	25% Normal Hb AA 50% Trait Hb AS 25% Disease Hb SS
6	Sickle Cell Trait Hb AS	Normal Hb AA	50% Trait Hb AS 50% Normal Hb AA
7	Sickle Cell Trait Hb AS	Hemoglobin C trait Hb AC	25% Trait Hb AS 25% Trait Hb AC 25% Normal Hb AA 25% Disease Hb SC
8	Sickle Cell Trait Hb AS	Beta Thalassemia Trait	25% Trait AS 25% Beta Thal Trait 25% Normal Hb AA 25% Disease S beta Thal

Your primary care doctor or specialist can direct you to a nearby university hospital. So can neighbors who are nurses or medical technicians, or friends who have already been down this road. You may also contact your state or county's medical society or any of the organizations listed in the "Resources" section at the end of this book for referrals to university hospitals.

THE PARENTS' OPTIONS

A counselor can help determine the odds, but only the parents can decide whether to bring into the world a child who may have severe symptoms and pain, and who may not live out a full lifespan.

Some couples would rather not risk having children who are likely to be born with sickle cell disease. Such a couple has three options:

- avoid pregnancy completely
- have the baby only when they know through prenatal tests that the fetus is perfectly healthy
- request pre-implantation genetic diagnosis. (Bloom, 1999, pp. 82-83)

As you will see, none of these options is without a sting.

AVOIDING PREGNANCY

Avoiding pregnancy is the simplest and least expensive option. It is also safest to the mother. A couple may naturally feel emotional pain knowing they can never have their own biological child.

Couples have several ways of avoiding pregnancy.

- Contraceptives, such as condoms or foams, are readily available at the local drug store. Remember that it takes only one incident of unprotected sex to impregnate a woman. Because the choices are difficult once the woman is pregnant, couples

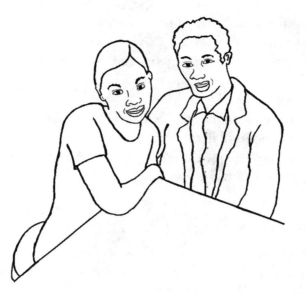

should talk frankly with one another about the importance of contraception.

- Another method of avoiding pregnancy is sterilization. The male can undergo a vasectomy, which is the tying of the tubes that allow sperm to move from the testes to the penis. The female may have her Fallopian tubes (the organs in which the eggs are fertilized) tied. Neither operation affects sexual performance. Both are usually, but not always, nonreversible.

ABORTING ALL BUT HEALTHY FETUSES

The second option is to have the baby *only* if tests determine that the fetus is healthy. This option may create new obstacles for the couple.

OBSTACLES TO ABORTION

One obstacle is religious. Abortion is prohibited by the Islamic religion as well as by the Roman Catholic Church. Many Protestant churches also discourage or forbid abortion. It is not permitted in Orthodox Judaism, with several exceptions.

Religion aside, many women—and of course many men as well—feel that it is morally wrong to abort the fetus at any stage of the pregnancy.

Legal restrictions on abortion may also pose difficulties. While abortion has been legal in all states for a quarter of a century, many states have recently placed restrictions on it. Ask your legal advisor about the abortion laws in your state.

PRE-IMPLANTATION GENETIC DIAGNOSIS

The third option for a couple that has decided not to risk having a child born with sickle cell disease is *"pre-implantation genetic diagnosis (PGD)."* PGD is an attractive option because it doesn't require parents to decide to abort the fetus if it will be born with sickle cell disease. This procedure involves taking eggs from the woman's ovary *before* she is pregnant and fertilizing them in a laboratory dish.

When the fertilized eggs begin to divide, one of the cells is taken out for DNA analysis and tested for sickle cell anemia or any other genetic disease. If the embryo is genetically normal, it is implanted into the mother, who completes the pregnancy.

PGD is highly experimental. At present, only thirty successful pregnancies have been accomplished using PGD. It is very costly, and is not easily accessible.

PROSPECTS FOR THE FUTURE

Today the genetic counselor's primary role is to

- provide information about genetic diseases and available resources
- predict the likelihood of a healthy baby
- inform the parents of the available options.

But tomorrow, the counselor might be able to do much more. Researchers in Durham, North Carolina, may have discovered a new method of gene therapy that corrects the defective sickle cell genes. (Clark, 1998, p.13) However, there are still many difficulties to overcome before this method can be used on humans.

DETECTION

The tests that diagnose birth defects, including sickle cell disease are:

AMNIOCENTESIS

Amniocentesis is performed (under local anesthesia) by inserting a large needle through the abdomen in order to withdraw a small amount of the amniotic fluid from the fetus. The sample fluid contains cells from the fetus that can be grown and whose DNA can then be analyzed.

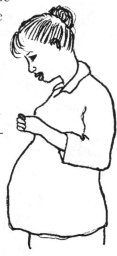

This procedure can be done only in the sixteenth through the eighteenth week of pregnancy, and the results take two to three weeks, which means that the woman will be well into the pregnancy before she can be tested and get results. Because the test must be done fairly late, the woman faces some risks, not only from an abortion, if she opts for one, but from the sampling procedure itself.

Another procedure for pre-natal diagnosis is chorionic villus sampling (CVS). This can be performed somewhat earlier, at twelve to fourteen weeks, and the results can be seen within forty-eight hours. However, the faster procedure carries 1%-2% greater risk of miscarriage. Further, the test is less accurate. This means there is a higher possibility that some women, on the basis of this test, might accidentally abort babies that would have been perfectly healthy.

NEWBORN SCREENING

Most states in the US now provide universal newborn screening for hemoglobin problems including sickle cell disease. If babies can be screened at birth, parents can be alerted to take preventive measures, like providing daily penicillin, a treatment that saves many lives.

If your baby is born in a hospital, blood tests are usually done in the newborn nursery. If you are not sure if your child was tested, have your child retested with the simple blood test called *the hemoglobin electrophoresis.*

SUMMING UP

The truths we wrestle with through genetic counseling can be bitter, but the nature of sickle cell disease requires that we think about them.

- Under certain conditions a man and a woman who love one another may be well advised not to have children.
- With all the other problems in your life, it is also important that you know your genetic map. That is the only way you can *decide* in good conscience whether to risk passing sickle cell trait and sickle cell disease down to the next generation.

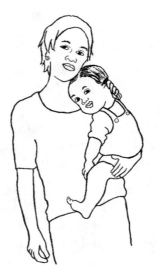

CHAPTER FOUR

Raising Children Who Have Sickle Cell Disease

Proverbs 22:6 Train a child in the way he should go, and when he is old he will not turn from it.

P arents whose children have sickle cell disease face special problems and pressures. In this chapter we'll talk about some of these. We'll also tell you how to work with your health care provider. Finally, we will make some suggestions about how to talk to your child.

WHAT'S REQUIRED OF THE PARENT

Parenting is the most rewarding job but it is also one of the toughest. Bringing up an African-American or minority youngster can be tougher still. While the opportunities are great for a minority child born today, the child also faces great dangers, from racism in the larger society and from the poverty, drugs, and violence that devastate many minority communities.

No wonder, then, that the parent of a child with a serious, long-term illness like sickle cell disease is often over-burdened. Look at what this disease requires of such a parent.

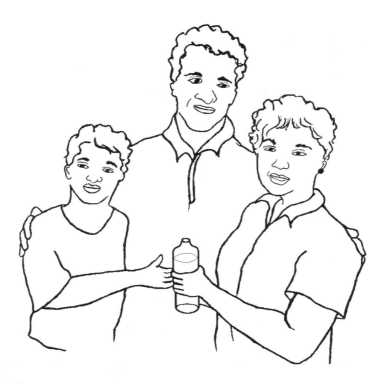

- First, you must become a student of the disease. That means you must get to know the preventive techniques available and how to get medical help when it is needed. It also means learning to recognize and treat potential problems before they get serious.
- Second, you must encourage your child's growth and independence without becoming overprotective.
- Finally, if you have more than one child, you must stretch yourself to give enough attention to your healthy children. Otherwise, they are likely to become jealous of the child with sickle cell disease.

In short, sickle cell disease calls on all the parents' wisdom and love.

Sometimes, it may seem to call on more than any one human

being could possibly have. Parents may feel that their own hold on ordinary life is slipping away. Careers can sink—because, just as your child is likely to experience long and frequent absences from school, you, as parent, may experience long and frequent absences from work to care for your child when he or she becomes ill.

This uncertainty may affect your choice of career, your ability to do your job well, and your chance to be promoted. Even if your company allows family leave, such policies often don't make up for lost job income.

Though family and friends often form a support community around those who suffer, parents facing their human burdens, day after day, may sometimes feel alone.

The fact is you are not alone. There are many public and private resources that can help you.

PARENTAL GUILT

Any parent who passes on to a child a genetic trait that makes it more likely the child will have a chronic illness is likely to feel guilty. Even if you, the parents, didn't know anything about the trait before you had the child, you may be stung by the knowledge that you *could* have known. *With appropriate genetic counseling, sickle cell disease is one hundred percent preventable.*

While prevention is possible it presents real life problems of its own. How do you ask the person you just fell in love with to show you his or her genetic map? For that matter, how much thought do most people give to how their genes might damage a child not yet conceived? As you struggle through the problems of an everyday African American life, such questions may seem far away.

Even people who seek genetic counseling before they plan a family will face emotional and spiritual problems that can become crises. Especially, they must struggle to decide whether to bring a child into the world, knowing that the child may suffer from sickle cell disease. Either decision one makes can cause guilt.

ONCE YOU KNOW THE LIKELY OUTCOMES

There are strong options for parents who have had genetic counseling, who know the likely outcomes, and who still want to have a child without sickle cell disease.

ADOPTION

Some parents choose to adopt a child. Giving a home to a child that otherwise may not have one can be as fulfilling as being the biological parent. There are many agencies that can help in this process.

IN VITRO FERTILIZATION

Couples who decide to have their own biologic children can do so by using in vitro fertilization. In this procedure, a sperm cell is introduced to an egg cell outside the body, in a test tube, rather than inside the body, in a Fallopian tube or in the womb. Because there is a 25 percent probability of a couple each with sickle cell trait having a child with sickle cell disease, the embryo is allowed to develop in the test tube until it is determined that it is free of major genetic problems, including sickle cell disease. The embryo is then implanted into the mother's womb.

The *Journal of the American Medical Association* featured a report of a couple in Detroit, each with sickle cell trait, who desired a child without sickle cell disease. The couple wanted to avoid the decision to abort an affected fetus. In vitro fertilization was used and the embryo was tested with DNA analysis. The embryo without sickle cell disease was implanted successfully.

In vitro fertilization is expensive. But even for those who can afford it, the issues it raises can't be taken lightly. For example, the procedure requires that more than one embryo be produced in order to ensure a successful and healthy implant. While some parents can make the "test tube solution" work for them, others, because of religious or other moral scruples, cannot because it requires them to authorize the destruction of unused "test tube" embryos.

We've been talking as if all pregnancies were planned, but of course that isn't the case. A frequent result of an unplanned pregnancy is that you may be raising your child as a single parent. It is hard enough to raise a healthy child alone. It is far more difficult to raise a child with sickle cell disease without another loving parent to share the tears, the anxieties, the emotional and financial burdens, as well as the joys and triumphs. That's why it's important for all people who carry the sickle cell trait to know how to prevent sickle cell disease.

But knowledge is of little value if we don't act on it. Let's listen to one couple hashing out their problem with friends. The couple is Derrick and Laquana, and they've just been told by their genetic counselor that they carry the sickle cell trait and that they have one chance in four of having a child with sickle cell disease. The other couple, Keeshawn and Shaniqua, haven't yet been tested but they plan to be. Laquana opens the discussion.

DERRICK AND LAQUANA'S STORY

Laquana. Derrick and I went to the doctor last week to get tested for sickle trait and other hemoglobin problems.

Derrick. Yeah, turns out we both have sickle trait.

Keeshawn. Have you decided what you'll do?

Laquana. We've thought it over a lot. Derrick wants a child, and says he's ready to be a really involved father. And you know, for me. . .well, we ladies do have that biological clock that keeps ticking. And I'm at the point in my career now where I can take some time off without risking my job. So we've decided to have a child.

Shaniqua. Congratulations! I'm scared about the possibility of having a child with sickle cell disease. It's hard enough to raise a normal child.

Derrick. We know it's no piece of cake. But from what the doctor told us and stuff we've been reading off the internet, the outlook for kids with sickle cell disease is a lot better than it used to be. There are new treatments, better ways to prevent crises, even occasional cures with bone marrow transplant, and a lot more support out there for families.

Shaniqua. You know me — I have to be blunt: I just don't think it's right to bring another child into the world with a chronic illness if we can help it.

Keeshawn. Yeah, that's my feeling too. Shaniqua and I have decided that when she gets pregnant, we'll have pre-natal testing. If the fetus tests positive for sickle cell disease, she'll have an abortion. It's not fair to bring a child into the world who's going to suffer so much, and who might have a shorter life after all that suffering.

Shaniqua. Yes. If we decide that we can't have a biological child, there are so many kids in the world who need a loving home. We can adopt one.

Laquana. Well, there you are. We feel that abortion is something we can't handle. Derrick and I will also have pre-natal testing, but if the fetus tests positive for sickle cell disease, we're going to use the rest of the pregnancy to learn as much as we can about the disease and that way give our child the longest, healthiest, happiest life possible.

Derrick. That's right. We know it won't be easy, but we've thought about it a lot. If the baby is born with sickle cell, she is going to get the best loving and caring any baby can get.

DERRICK AND LAQUANA HAVE THEIR CHILD

Derrick and Laquana went through with the plan they talked about. Throughout Laquana's pregnancy, she was carefully monitored by the pediatrician. Now the baby, Booker, is three months old and has sickle cell disease type SS. At their pediatrician's recommendation, they regularly see a pediatric hematologist at

University Medical Center. They're very happy with her. Derrick and Laquana bring her their questions and she takes time to explain things.

SUPPORT AND NETWORKING

As long as children with sickle cell disease do come into the world, they deserve to get the best, most loving care. By drawing on the education, support, and networking other people can provide, parents can anticipate problems and deal with them before they get too big.

One of a parent's first obligations is to know what to expect at each stage of a child's illness and so recognize problems at their earliest stages, when they can be dealt with most effectively. Managing a disease means knowing the best ways to avoid a serious outbreak of symptoms or still more serious complications. Knowing what to expect, not being caught off guard, means the parent can react earlier, in a calmer frame of mind, and prevent some emergencies.

DERRICK AND LAQUANA FIND SUPPORT

Let's tune in on Derrick and Laquana again and see what they're up to now that their son Booker is nine months old. They are talking with their family physician.

Laquana: Booker's first crisis really shook me up. Even though we were ready for it and he got great care, he was so helpless.

Dr. Watkins: I hear what you're saying, Laquana. And I'm sorry that, the way things happened, you and Derrick had to go through it without the emotional help you might have had. Now let's correct that.

Remember a few months ago I told you that we have a sickle cell parents' support group here at the University. Over the years I've found that it really helps to talk about your experiences, fears,

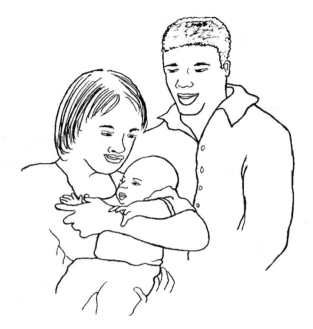

and solutions with other folks going through the same process. You'll meet regularly and exchange phone numbers and e-mails. Please give it some thought.

Derrick: That sounds interesting. Feeling isolated is part of the problem. I don't mean you doctors aren't helping. But sometimes we just need to talk about our feelings and our uncertainty with people who are going through what we're going through.

Dr. Watkins: I can understand that. I think you'll find what you're looking for in the parents' groups. What they do is share information. Someone will give you tips about something that's worked for them in dealing with a child who's hurting and scared and discouraged.

And I'm not just talking about physical pain and illness. Before long Booker will be in school. He'll want to run around with the other kids, he'll want to feel sharp in class. But there will be days when he can't run around; days when it's all he can do to hold his head off his desk. Other parents can tell you how they've been able to reassure their own children, and what they've said to teachers that helps.

Both of you will need comfort and counsel yourselves. You'll worry about medical expenses and about time lost from work. Talking with people who have found solutions, or at least ways of living with tough situations—no question but that helps.

Sometimes you'll come away from these meetings with a new piece of information—the name of an agency or a doctor someone thinks highly of, or of a treatment plan that's worked. There's no end to the resources caring people come up with when they put their heads together to solve common problems. I'm looking forward to hearing what you have to say about the group you join. I feel pretty confident you'll agree it's one of the best tips I've given you.

TALKING TO YOUR CHILD

The most common problem your child may have is pain. When your child is old enough to understand, talk to him or her about telling you when it hurts. Love, hugs, and reassurance go a long way to quiet fears. There will be a day when your child will want to know why he or she is different from other children. That is the time to begin the life-long journey of teaching your child about sickle cell. Denying, minimizing, ignoring, and running away from the facts will only hurt your child in the long run. Learn all you can so you can fill your child with life saving knowledge. Tell your child about the blood cells. Show pictures and drawings the child can relate to. Tell your child why it's so important to drink a lot of water, keep warm in cold weather, cool in hot weather, and how not to become over-tired. Encourage your child with play, games that challenge the mind, and reading. Limit television time and encourage reading. Talk about careers that challenge the mind and don't strain the body.

Teaching your child openly and honestly to talk to you about pain

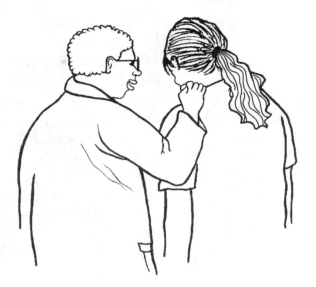

is essential. If that communication is managed well, your child won't complain of pain in order to avoid school, homework, or chores.

Let your child know that he or she will have lots of help in being his or her best, and will have a full life ahead—as long as it is thoughtfully prepared for. There will be some stormy days, to be sure, but if the atmosphere is honest and informed, there will be far more sunny ones.

Partner with your child's health care providers to learn what to discuss with your child. These specialists may offer tips, books, pictures, videos and other materials that will make teaching fun and understandable.

Be an example for your child. What you do and how you act has a greater impact than what you say. Children follow your footsteps. If they see you calling in sick to work when you have other plans, they will repeat the pattern and use the disease as an excuse to avoid school or other responsibilities. *Be an example of responsibility, caring, giving, and hope.* This will speak volumes to your child and you will see the seeds you have planted come to bloom in your child's life.

Take time to have family fun with outings, trips, and activities. It is critical to have the child with sickle cell disease fit into the family unit and not have the other siblings become resentful or neglected.

FINANCING YOUR CHILD'S CARE

Medical costs can be huge for a child with sickle cell disease. Most of the treatment programs we've talked about include social workers who will help you plan the best way to finance your child's care.

Programs like Medicaid, available to poor people in all states and territories of the United States, as well as Puerto Rico and Washington, D.C., can pay for practically all of your child's medical care if you qualify. The specific requirements an individual or family must meet to qualify for Medicaid vary from state to state. The best source of information on your state's requirements is a social worker or the local Medicaid office.

Medicaid's stated policy now is to try to eventually force most subscribers into Medicaid-HMO's, but patients or their parents can apply for exemptions, which are usually granted, in the case of serious, chronic illnesses, like sickle cell disease.

For those who earn too much to qualify for Medicaid but who do not have insurance coverage, the options may narrow to community or county hospitals and health care centers. These facilities can have excellent care. Seek those hospitals affiliated with medical schools and teaching programs. This is where some of the best treatment is available. The fact is, help is available. If you don't find it at first keep looking. You will find it eventually.

CHAPTER 5

Sickle Cell Disease

THE TYPES OF HEMOGLOBINS THAT CAUSE SICKLE CELL DISEASE

Sickle cell disease is a family of hemoglobin combinations, including

- hemoglobin SS (called sickle cell anemia)
- SC
- S beta Thalassemia
- SD Punjab
- SO Arab
- SE
- SS (hereditary persistence of fetal hemoglobin).

All of these combinations have sickle complications, but some are more severe than others. There are many genetic differences within these hemoglobin combinations that we still do not fully understand that make some have a milder course and some a more severe course.

HEMOGLOBIN SS—SICKLE CELL ANEMIA

Sickle Cell Anemia, or Hb SS, is caused by inheriting two sickle genes, one from each parent. This is the most common type of sickle cell disease.

Symptoms may include moderate to severe anemia, increased infections, tissue damage, organ damage and recurrent pain episodes. The anemia is generally well tolerated by patients but does lead to premature gall stones in many. The anemia may become life-threatening during aplastic crises or splenic sequestration crises. Treatment with blood transfusions may be needed. Removal of the spleen is done for splenic sequestration in older children when it happens over and over.

Children and some adults may have increased bacterial infections. Tissue damage may cause pain and scarring. Strokes may occur in children because of blocked blood flow to the brain. The blocked blood flow to bone may cause pain episodes, and lead to aseptic necrosis of the hip and shoulder bones. Blockage of the eye blood vessels may lead to bleeding into the eye and loss of vision. As patients age, damage to the lungs and kidneys can cause breathing problems and inability to filter toxins from the blood. Pain episodes can be unpredictable and disruptive to normal life.

HEMOGLOBIN SC

Those with Hb SC disease, the second most common type of sickle cell disease, inherit a Hb C gene from one parent and a Hb S gene from the other. In general, those with Hb SC have a sickle syndrome which is very similar to sickle cell anemia, though the hemolysis is usually less severe so the anemia is milder. The reported average life expectancy of those with Hb SC is in the mid-60s compared to the mid-40s for those with Hb SS. There is less incidence of stroke compared to Hb SS. Having an enlarged spleen is much more common in older children and adults, though it doesn't work very well to fight infections. This can lead to splenic sequestration, or the swelling of the spleen, with sickled red blood cells later in life. There may be more eye problems that require yearly eye examinations and sometimes preventive laser surgery. Bone damage, such as AVN, or avascular necrosis of the hip and shoulder bones, is also more common. Other symptoms are similar to Hb SS.

HEMOGLOBIN S BETA THALASSEMIA

Beta thalassemias are inherited disorders of Beta globin production, a part of the hemoglobin molecule. In most people, the molecule's blueprint structure is normal but the rate of production is reduced. The problem is in the communication between the blueprint DNA and the manufacturing plant. Decreased hemoglobin production causes smaller than normal red blood cells, which look like bull's eye targets under the microscope. Beta thalassemia can combine with the sickle hemoglobin to cause sickle beta thalassemia, the third most common type of sickle cell disease.

Sickle beta thalassemia comes in two types, Sickle beta 0 thalassemia and sickle beta + thalassemia.

The severity of the problems related to Beta thalassemia is unpredictable. Most people with Sickle Beta+ thalassemia have working spleens and fewer problems with infection, fewer pain episodes, and less organ damage. The prognosis is usually good.

Those with Sickle Beta 0 thalassemia may have very severe disease, identical to sickle cell anemia or Hb SS. Hemoglobin levels may be higher on average. Spleens stop working later in childhood, and enlargement of the spleen is common into adulthood. Pain episodes, organ damage, and prognosis may be similar or perhaps even worse for bone and eye problems when compared to sickle cell anemia Hb SS.

Genetic counseling and prenatal diagnosis for sickle cell,

should always consider that one partner may be a carrier of a beta thalassemia gene. These carriers are easily missed because their hemoglobin levels may be normal or near normal.

HEMOGLOBIN SD, SO, SE

There are D hemoglobins that interact with Hb S, causing milder sickle cell disease with occasional pain episodes.

Hemoglobin O-Arab has significance in sickle cell disease because it interacts with Hb S to produce clinical symptoms like Hb SS disease.

Hb SE sickle cell disease is rare with only five reported cases. These cases were all mild. The Hb E gene is very common in many areas of Southeast Asia, India, and China.

HEMOGLOBIN SS- HPFH OR HEREDITARY PERSISTENCE OF FETAL HEMOGLOBIN

Hemoglobin F (fetal hemoglobin) is the main hemoglobin in the baby's red blood cells before birth. Fetal hemoglobin declines over the first six months of life to near adult levels. This decline may be slower in those with sickle syndromes. People with Beta thalassemias usually have high levels for life. Those with sickle cell anemia have levels from 2% to 20% with some evidence that those with higher levels have less complications. The preventive medication hydroxyurea increases fetal hemoglobin levels.

HOW SICKLE CELL DISEASE SHOWS ITSELF

People with sickle cell disease have hemoglobin that is different in only one way from that of the normal population. This simple difference is the basis for all the problems that result from sickle cell disease.

The difference is *sickle hemoglobin*, which makes the red blood cells rigid. When sickle hemoglobin loses its oxygen, it forms rigid, crystal-like rods called polymers. It is these rods inside the red blood cells that cause them to take on a sickle shape. Clumping of these sickled red blood cells leads to blockage of blood vessels. And this blockage of blood flow (ischemia) causes tissue death (infarction) and pain.

Sickle red blood cells are stickier than non sickle ones. This also causes blocked blood flow. Platelets, the cells that plug up cuts and cause clotting to occur, become too active and cause clotting in blood vessels that aren't cut—which stops blood flow. All of these actions lead to sickle cell pain episodes.

Some crises are sudden, severe, and others are not. Pain episodes can be caused by low oxygen, infections, dehydration, overheating, cold exposure, your period (menses), and stress.

A newborn with sickle cell disease does not show any signs of it until six months of age. The first symptom of the disorder in infants is usually swelling of the hands and feet (hand-foot syndrome or *acute sickle dactylitis*). This is caused by blocked blood flow, which is caused by sickled red blood cells. This results in a rapid, painful swelling of the bone marrow cavity of the small bones in the hands and feet.

The way it works is this. When sickle hemoglobin (Hgb S) loses the oxygen it is carrying, it clumps into long chains. This causes the shape of the red blood cell to become rigid and sickle like, and makes it hard for the red blood cell to pass through the tiny blood tubing called *capillaries*, which are actually narrower than the red blood cells. These sticky, rigid red blood cells cling to the smallest blood vessels, causing them to become blocked. Over time, low blood flow in these narrowed blood vessels causes the tissue to die. Tissue death in turn causes swelling and pain. Pain in itself stim-

ulates more blood vessel narrowing, further reducing blood flow and triggering a chain reaction of the sickling cycle. The hard red blood cells break apart earlier than normal.

THE IMPORTANCE OF READING THE SIGNS

Nothing is more important for patients and families than to recognize the symptoms of sickle cell disease early.

Many of the symptoms mimic those of other diseases whose treatment can be quite different. For instance,

- Abdominal pain, in a sickle cell patient, might seem to be the usual pain episode related to the disease; it might, however, be due to gall bladder stones—a condition known as *biliary colic*.
- Bone pain in a person with sickle cell disease may be mistaken for a typical pain episode, and the patient or family may first try pain medication at home. On the other hand, that pain could be caused by a serious bone infection known as *osteomyelitis*, which requires different treatment.

In order to deal effectively with sickle cell disease you should be able to:

- recognize the typical features of a sickle cell patient
- recognize the early signs in a previously healthy baby.
- know when to seek urgent medical attention.
- learn to anticipate and understand the differences in appearance and development between children or siblings with sickle cell anemia and others without the disease.

Because thickening of the blood may occur anywhere in the body and cause blockages of the blood vessels, sickle cell anemia can affect a wide range of body systems. That is why complications of the disease can vary so much. Symptoms that result from any of these complications are most severe during periods called "sickle cell crisis."

Table 2
Here are some of the problems that can occur:

Diagnosis	Reason for symptoms	Symptoms
Acute Chest Syndrome	Lack of blood flow to the lungs	Shortness of breath, chest pain.
Anemia	Breakdown of blood, lack of production	Weakness, tiredness, pale color, swelling in feet, shortness of breath, fainting
Infections	Damage to the spleen	Fever, severe headaches and neck pain, chest pains.
Priapism	Lack of blood flow from the penis	Prolonged and painful erection
Stroke	Lack of blood flow to brain or bleeding within the brain.	Headache, weakness, numbness, paralysis, slurred speech or dizziness.
Bone Infarction	Lack of blood supply to the bone	Severe prolonged bone pain
Splenic Sequestration	Sickle cells become trapped in the spleen	Stomach pain, swelling, weakness, tiredness, pale in color
Leg Ulcers	Lack of blood supply to the skin	Skin ulcers that are slow to heal
Gall Stones	Make more bile stones from red blood cells breaking apart	Stomach pain, nausea, vomiting, can not eat greasy foods
Pain Episode	Blocked blood flow to muscles and bones	Pain in the arms, legs and back typical of past episodes
Growth and Puberty Delay	Increased calories needed	Short height, late signs of puberty
Vision— Eye problems	Damage to blood vessels in the eye	Loss of vision, flashing lights
Swelling of Hands and	Sickle cells blocking blood flow	Painful swelling of feet and hands

PHYSICAL ISSUES

Generally, a child's final height is not affected by sickle cell disease, but the rate of growth during childhood and adolescence is slower. So final height may not be reached until the early twenties. Weight tends to be abnormally low. Bone development is delayed. Sexual maturation takes longer, causing delayed development and onset of a period in females and delayed maturation of males' sexual organs. In severe cases of delayed growth and development, hormonal therapy may help to reverse the problem.

PSYCHOSOCIAL ISSUES

Psychosocial issues such as depression, low self-esteem, poor family relationships, and social isolation can arise from being chronically ill. School grades may be lower, if students miss many days of class. Chronic pain is a part of these childrens' lives but others sometimes misinterpret such students' reaction to pain as addictive drug-seeking behavior, or slacking off. Some patients will become addicted to pain medications. It is important to have good family support, group support, and medical care to help you with all the issues that you will face.

ECONOMIC ISSUES

The economic impact of sickle cell disease is enormous. Patients can require hospitalization for acute pain crisis, aplastic anemia, stroke, acute chest syndrome, infections and even priapism. During hospitalization, patients will often need blood transfusions, intravenous fluid therapy, and pain management.

Careful outpatient evaluation, management, and prevention can help curb some of the cost of hospitalization. Antibiotics and immunizations can be given in the first years of life to help minimize infections. Rehabilitative services may also be required.

INFECTIONS

Infections are one of the greatest dangers to those with sickle cell disease. Bacterial infections are the most common cause of death in children during the first five years of life. Although those under three are at greatest risk for life threatening infections, they can be gotten at any age. Because the spleen doesn't work properly there is a decreased ability to fight off overwhelming infection. The spleen is the body's major defense against deadly germs. Serious infections such as blood infections (sepsis), infection surrounding the brain (meningitis), and lung infection (pneumonia) caused by germs are common. The bones and joints may also become infected.

Infections of the bladder and kidney are more common among people with sickle cell disease. These infections may also be more severe. Lives can be saved by finding these infections early and treating them with the proper antibiotic. See the section on medications within this chapter for more on this topic.

PREVENTION OF PROBLEMS: FARMS

The best way to avoid problems is to prevent them from happening. Remember FARMS—the basic principles of prevention:

F—is for Fluids and Fever. Drink plenty of water and manage fever. If you get a fever see your health care provider right away.

A—is for Air. Make sure you get enough oxygen, especially in unpressurized airplanes.

R—is for Rest. Get plenty of sleep, do not over do it, and take plenty of breaks when your body feels tired.

M—is for prevention Medications, like daily penicillin for children under six or hydrea for pain prevention. The vitamin Folate is needed to make new red blood cells.

S—is for Situations to avoid, like getting too hot or cold, avoiding smoking, alcohol or illegal drugs.

Exercise and work outdoors wearing the proper clothing for the season. Drink plenty of water, and take frequent rest and water breaks. Carry a water bottle with you and drink from it often. Avoid swimming pools that are too cold or hot tubs that are too hot.

Avoid emotional stress by pacing projects and work. Avoid situations that you know are upsetting. Join a support group that offers spiritual and emotional support.

FLUIDS

The simple act of consuming extra water can dramatically delay the sickling effect. Even a little bit of water can make a tremendous difference—drinking 10 percent more water, for example, can slow down sickling by 1,700 percent.

It is especially important for children with sickle cell to drink plenty of water because kidneys—along with all the other organs— are damaged by sickle cells. Once damaged, the kidneys cannot help the body retain water very well. Loss of water through urine continues at a high rate all day and all night. It is very easy for people with sickle cell to quickly become dehydrated if they do not drink enough to replace the water lost.

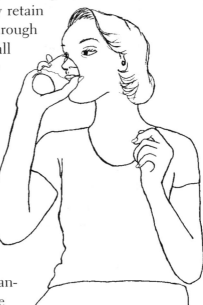

The best fluid is *water*. Other fluids like juice, milk, soup, fruit, or sports drinks are also fine to add some varia- tion, as are popsicles. On the other hand, drinks with *caffeine* (cola, coffee), alcohol, or methylxan- thine found in iced or hot tea are not a good idea. These ingredients make the kidney release more water into the urine. If your child is fond of cola or tea, try to limit her to no more than two glasses a day.

The amount of water you need to drink depends on your size. What pediatricians call the maintenance rate of fluids is the minimum you need to avoid dehydration. Half again this amount is even better.

Table 3 (page 48) indicates how much an individual child should drink. Drinking more than the amount shown is fine, and may be necessary when the child is ill, exercising, or hot. In particular, when having sickle cell pain, make sure that he or she drinks at least the higher of the recommended amounts.

A I R

Air means getting enough air—and oxygen—into your lungs and into your red blood cells. The red blood cells, with sickle hemoglobin, sickle when the hemoglobin gives up its oxygen. The ways to rob the red cells of oxygen include: smoking, mountain climbing, having asthma or pneumonia, and flying in unpressurized aircraft.

You should not smoke, and if you do, you should stop. Smoking damages lungs and robs the body of valuable oxygen. Family members who smoke should do so outside, and away from, the one with sickle cell disease. Asthma can be treated with medications that open the airways and prevent them from closing. Symptoms of shortness of breath, fever, cough, or chest pain may all be early signs of pneumonia or chest syndrome. If you have any of these see your doctor immediately for a complete evaluation. Do not go to higher altitudes in aircraft or hike on mountains without taking oxygen along. (See the section on air travel.)

Table 3
Metric units version

Body weight weight (kg)	recommended range per day (liters)
5	0.5 to 0.7
10	1 to 1.4
15	1.2 to 1.8
20	1.4 to 2.2
25	1.5 to 2.3
30	1.7 to 2.5
35	1.8 to 2.7
45	2 to 3
55	2.3 to 3.4
65	2.5 to 3.8
75	2.8 to 4.1

English units version

Body weight (pounds)	recommended range per day (8 ounce cups)
10	2 to 3 cups
25	4 to 6 cups
30	5 to 8 cups
45	6 to 9 cups
55	7 to 10 cups
75	8 to 11 cups
100	9 to 13 cups
130	10 to 15 cups
150	11 to 17 cups
175	12 to 18 cups

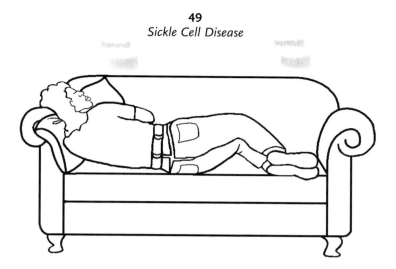

REST

Exercising to exhaustion makes the body chemistry change to a state called *lactic acidosis*. Acidosis will often trigger sickle cell pain, and a child with a lower blood count level will reach this state sooner than one with a higher level.

To avoid exhaustion, children with sickle cell should take frequent breaks when playing. During vigorous play, taking a break every 15 to 20 minutes both to rest and to drink usually will allow them to continue their activities without developing lactic acidosis. One young man, for example, often developed sickle cell pain if he played basketball for 30 minutes straight. However, he found that he could cut down on his pain episodes by playing the first quarter of a basketball game, resting the second quarter, playing the third, and resting the fourth. Physical education teachers or coaches may need a note from the family or doctor to explain this situation.

MEDICATIONS AND MEDICAL CARE

Sickle cell patients should be under the care of a medical team that understands sickle cell disease. All newborn babies with sickle cell disease should be placed on daily penicillin to prevent serious infections. All of the childhood immunizations should be given plus the pneumococcal vaccine. Parents should know how to check for a fever because this signals the possibility of serious infection. The following are general guidelines to keep the sickle cell patient healthy:

1. Take the vitamin folic acid (folate) daily to help make new red cells
2. Take daily penicillin until age six to prevent serious infection
3. Drink plenty of water daily (8-10 glasses for adults)
4. Avoid extremes of temperatures
5. Avoid over-exertion and stress
6. Get plenty of rest
7. Get regular checkups from expert health care providers

Patients and families should watch for the following conditions that need an urgent medical evaluation:

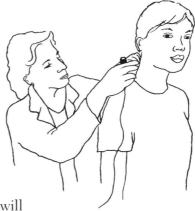

1. Fever
2. Chest pain
3. Shortness of breath
4. Increasing tiredness
5. Abdominal swelling
6. Unusual headache
7. Any sudden weakness or loss of feeling
8. Pain that will not go away with home treatment
9. Priapism (painful erection that will not go down)
10. Sudden vision change

SITUATIONS

Being either chilled or overheated changes the blood flow patterns in the body and can lead to sickle cell pain. When the weather is cold, dress your child warmly. When the weather is hot and she's spending time outside, make sure she takes frequent breaks in the shade or an air-conditioned room. Many people find that swimming in unheated water can chill the body quickly and trigger sickle cell pain. That's why children with sickle cell should take rest breaks often to dry off and warm up.

When the weather is changing quickly or your activities will take you from the hot outdoors to cool air-conditioning, make sure to dress your child in layers so that you can help regulate her temperature. A sweatsuit or warm-up outfit can be very helpful for staying warm before and after exercise.

Avoid using illegal drugs such as cocaine that are deadly to those without sickle cell disease and many times more deadly for those with it. Alcohol should also be avoided because it dehydrates the body and makes the blood more acid—just the right conditions to increase sickling.

IMMUNIZATIONS

Because infections often trigger pain and other sickle cell crises, it is vitally important that you get immunized against certain preventable serious infections. Recommended immunizations include:

- pneumococcal (a common cause of pneumonia)
- influenza vaccine
- Hemophilus influenzae type B (a common cause of sore throats, sinus and middle ear infections, acute bronchitis, and pneumonia)
- meningococcus (a common cause of meningitis)

Immunizations should be given only when patients are in the best possible health. Immunizations should not be given when a sniffle, cold, or "flu" is present because then immunizations will more likely cause an unpleasant, or possibly dangerous, reaction. They may also be less effective.

Immunizations, should, if possible, be given when the patient

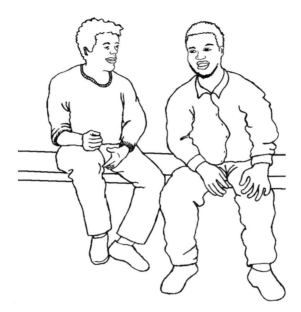

is young, before much damage to the spleen has occurred. Early detection and aggressive treatment of infection is key to preventing and/or reducing the severity of sickle crises.

PNEUMOCOCCAL VACCINE

The pneumococcal vaccine offers protection against 90% of the strains that cause serious infection in the United States. A new vaccine, Prevnar™, can be given as early as two months after birth followed by two more doses six to eight weeks apart and a booster dose at twelve months. This is followed by the Pneumovax™ at age two and five years.

MENINGOCOCCAL VACCINE

The meningococcal vaccine protects against a broad range of meningococcus strains. If you've had close contacts with patients having documented meningococcal infection be sure to check with your doctor, who may recommend a meningococcal immunization.

Patients travelling to areas where meningococcal disease is epidemic (check with your airport's travel clinic or with the Center for Disease Control's website, at www.cdc.gov/) should also receive one dose of the vaccine before leaving.

Household contacts of patients with meningococcal infection are at increased risk of infection themselves and should receive preventive treatment with the antibiotic rifampin.

For those who are unable to tolerate rifampin, there are several alternative antibiotics:

- ciprofloxaxin
- orofloxacin
- ceftriaxone—for pregnant women or children under twelve years old

Immunization for meningococcal infection is recommended not only for those who live with infected persons. It is also recommended for anyone who has had close contact with an infected patient in settings such as

- nursery schools
- day care centers
- camps

or for anyone who has had oral contact with an infected patient, such as kissing, mouth to mouth resuscitation, or sharing of the same utensil, plate, glass, cup, or toothbrush.

MALARIA PREVENTION

The prevention of malaria is complex and still controversial. What you can do for yourself is to avoid being bitten by the common Anopheles mosquito, which carries the disease.

Measures you can take:

- avoid travel, if possible, to areas where malaria is common
- avoid being outdoors in such areas at peak mosquito feeding times (dusk and dawn)
- use insect repellent regularly in such areas (increased dietary garlic and brewer's yeast have been described as excellent natural additional insect repellants)
- wear long pants and long sleeves in endemic areas (admittedly tough in the hot tropical and subtropical areas where malaria is common)
- use window screens.
- use bed netting treated with the chemical permethrin (recently shown to reduce malaria deaths in Africa)

For more detailed information about malaria, see the appendix.

LIFE EXPECTANCY

The most current information available from scientific articles is listed, and is the information we use. But keep in mind that the life expectancy keeps going up with newer treatments, better prevention, more education, genetics, healthy living, and good health care. In the Georgia Comprehensive Sickle Cell Center, we see

Table 4

Median survival of individuals of all ages with sickle cell disease based on sickle cell disease type and sex:

Sex and Genotype	Median Survival
Males with Hb SS	42 years
Females with Hb SS	48 years
Males with Hb SC	60 years
Females with Hb SC	68 years

several patients in their 50s, 60s, and 70s. We even have a 90 year old who drops in for monitoring and treatment.

Patients should be encouraged to live every day to the fullest and prepare for a life into adulthood. Preparation should be made for work, marriage, hobbies, and meaningful contributions to society. Our patient population includes lawyers, teachers, computer programmers, artists, moms, and dads.

MYTHS EXPLODED

Myth: Sickle cell is like a cold and you can catch it from someone with the disease.

Truth: You can not catch sickle cell disease, it is genetic. Only people who are born with this genetic defect can have it. It is life-long and is present at birth.

Myth: You must be Black to have sickle cell disease.

Truth: Sickle cell is a disease that affects people of all different racial and ethnic backgrounds, including African, Arabian, Israeli, Greek, Italian, Hispanic, Turkish, and Pakistani. The national poster child for sickle cell disease one year was a blond, blue-eyed Caucasian girl. All newborns should be screened at birth for hemoglobin traits and disease.

Myth: If our child has the disease, it means that she got the sickle cell gene from both my spouse and me.

Truth: This is true of sickle cell anemia, HbSS, but there are other types in which only one parent has passed on the sickle cell gene and the other has passed on a gene for another type of anemia, such as Hb C, D, E, O or thalassemia, that combine to produce sickle cell disease. This trait may be unknown to the partner.

Myth: Sickle cell trait is not important, it doesn't do anything.

Truth: Although it is a rare occurrence, sickle cell trait can cause bleeding in the urine. And under extremely severe conditions—at the limits of human endurance, such as military training or exercise at high altitude, for example—people with the trait can develop the same health problems as someone with sickle cell disease. Also, when your child grows up, if she and her spouse both have sickle cell trait, they should be aware that their children could be born with sickle cell disease.

Myth: People with sickle cell disease or sickle cell trait cannot get malaria.

Truth: People with sickle cell disease can get malaria, and may even have a worse case. However, people with sickle cell trait tend to survive malaria better than those without the trait.

Myth: People with sickle cell will not live past teenage years.

Truth: People with sickle cell now have a life expectancy at least into their mid 40s, thanks to several recent advances in care—in particular, new methods for preventing infections and treating fever.

Early detection of sickle cell through newborn screenings also improves survival from lung and spleen problems.

The first effective medication to improve sickle cell (hydroxyurea) recently was approved by the Food and Drug Administration.

Myth: There is no cure for sickle cell disease.

Truth: Over one hundred sickle cell patients in the United States have been cured by bone marrow transplant. The problem is this procedure needs a bone marrow donation from a genetically matched brother or sister. One must have enough complications from the disease to take the risk of the bone marrow transplant.

Myth: Sickle cell patients and their families cannot chart their own destiny.

Truth: Patients and families need to strike a balance between completely denying the presence of the disease, and living in a bubble. Learning about preventive measures and applying them can prevent complications and pain.

Myth: I have sickle cell trait, I can not donate blood

Truth: For nearly all purposes, blood with sickle trait is OK. The Blood Bank only tests for sickle trait upon request by the doctors ordering the blood for transfusion. There are uncommon situations where the presence of any sickle hemoglobin might cause problems (such as extensive transfusions for a patient with sickle cell disease, making it hard to test how much of the blood is the patient's own and how much is transfused blood).

Myth: My child has hemoglobin SC, this is the same as sickle cell trait.

Truth: Hemoglobin SC is very definitely a type of sickle cell disease, and it has symptoms. Painful episodes for a population of children with HbSC may not be as severe or frequent as in HbSS (homozygous sickle cell disease), but there is wide variation between individuals. After childhood, the complications of HbSC patients increase so that the disease becomes approximately similar in severity to adults with HbSS. Sickle cell pain typically involves bones (including joints and skull), but can affect nearly any part of the body.

In older school-age children and adolescents with HbSC, there is a high rate of two complications of sickle cell disease: damage to the joints (due to sickle cells interfering with blood flow to the heads of the femur and humerus), and damage to the retina of the eye (due to blocked blood vessels and abnormal growth of fragile new vessels that can bleed spontaneously). We routinely check HbSC children for these problems, and recommend annual retinal examination by an ophthalmologist after age 8. Other sickle cell complications are less frequent in HbSC than HbSS (stroke, acute lung problems, aplastic crisis) but can occur.

CLIMATE

There are some reports that the mild climate of the tropics may benefit sickle cell patients. It is known that exposure to extreme cold or hot temperatures can promote sickling. Proper clothing and protection from the temperature is necessary in climates that have temperature extremes. In dry climates, drinking a lot of water is important to keep up with water losses.

SPORTS

We encourage activities that require concentration and skill rather than endurance. Golf, martial arts, skateboarding, bowling, table tennis, and fencing are all good choices. Swimming in a heated pool is also recommended because of its low impact on the hip joints. "Extreme" or endurance sports (long distance competitive racing, for example), which push the body to exhaustion and cause dehydration, are likely to cause problems. Sports that involve cold temperatures (skiing, sky diving) or low oxygen (mountain climbing) will probably trigger sickle cell pain.

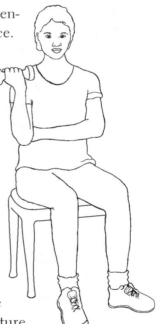

Common triggers for increased sickle cell pain are dehydration, temperature extremes (both cold and heat), low oxygen, exhaustion (lactic acidosis), infection, and stress. Sickle cell pains show up in certain places in the body because of vaso-occlusion. Generally, pain affects the long bones, the vertebrae, and the shin.

Active youngsters need to pay particular attention to the hip, where avascular necrosis is extremely common in young adults with sickle cell. This can be accelerated by repetitive injury from high-impact sports. Pain in the hip or knee should be evaluated by an orthopedist with sickle cell experience. Patients with diagnosed avascular necrosis of the hip should not participate in sports that involve repetitive jumping (basketball, dance, and gymnastics, to name a few) that may cause further injury to the hip joint.

Hydration before and during sports activity is critical. Rest breaks every 20 minutes to avoid acidosis should be scheduled.

For sprains and strains, avoid using ice. Try instead applying a cool, not cold, compress to reduce the risk of vasoconstriction, which can aggravate pain in the area.

If the patient has a very enlarged spleen, contact sports (football, hockey, lacrosse, etc.) present a risk of rupturing the organ, but the level of danger depends on the level of sports competition. Most elementary-school-age children can't hit hard enough to actually damage the spleen.

AIR TRAVEL

In some patients, sickle pain episodes are caused by flying. The major problem is a decrease in oxygen in the cabin air. The aircraft is only pressurized to about 7,000 feet, which is low enough to get some people with sickle cell in trouble. The other problem is related to dehydration. The humidity in the aircraft is very low and fluid intake needs to be markedly increased before and during the flight.

If you have had trouble flying, we would recommend supplemental oxygen at 2 liters per minute or 120 liters/hour. Most airlines are willing to provide this but require two weeks notice and a doctor's letter that establishes the need for oxygen and specifies the rate of flow.

Ask the airline for an aisle seat and plan to drink a pint of water an hour during the flight. You may wish to carry on the water you will need.

Takeoff and landing are not the critical times. The period of concern is when the plane is at greater than 10,000 feet because that is when the cabin pressure is reduced and supplementary oxygen will be needed by the person with sickle cell.

When travelling, make sure you have a supply of all of the medicines you will need during your trip. You also should have a letter from your doctor that summarizes your disease complications and your most recent laboratory results, so that, if illness occurs, the treating doctors will know average values. Be sure all vaccinations are up to date.

HEALTHY DIET, "NATURAL TREATMENTS"

While everyone needs to think about what they eat, a healthy diet is even more important for children with sickle cell disease. These key principles are good to follow:

- Children with sickle cell have the same basic nutritional requirements as anyone else.
- The food pyramid developed by the federal government is a useful guide.
- A healthy diet helps every child grow well and avoid illness.
- Learning and practicing good eating habits while still young can help prevent many diseases later in life, such as heart disease, cancer, stroke, and diabetes.
- So far, researchers believe that the same antioxidants and anti-clotting foods that help prevent heart disease, stroke, and cancer also help reduce health problems caused by sickle cell disease.
- Extra fluids are very important. Avoiding dehydration is a good way to decrease the likelihood of pain crises.

Recent research shows that children with sickle cell need more calories than other children, probably 20 percent more at rest. Extra calories are required because of the extra energy needed to make new red blood. The calories contained in our food are con-

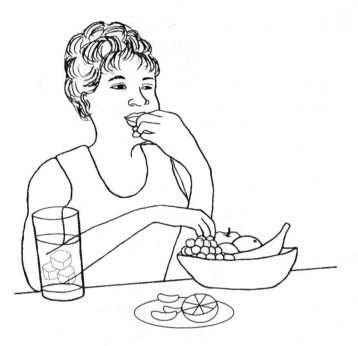

verted by our bodies into energy that is used to help us grow, ward off infection, and do our daily activities. Not getting enough calories may lead to delays in growth and maturation.

Be sure your child snacks on healthy foods, such as fruits, vegetables, and grains, not just junk food. Work in some additional calories (and protein) by putting peanut butter on celery or carrots; adding cheese, nuts, or wheat germ to appropriate foods; making milkshakes or yogurt smoothies; and serving pudding or instant breakfast drinks.

Even though children with sickle cell need more calories, it is just as important for them to maintain a normal weight. Obesity can lead to faster onset of *avascular necrosis of the hip,* where the hip bone loses its blood supply and collapses.

Constipation may be an unfortunate side effect of some of the medications required for the treatment of sickle cell pain. Consuming plenty of fiber, such as that found in whole grains and fruits, will help prevent or treat constipation. When opiates are used on a daily basis, you may need a stool softener as well as a high fiber diet. You must drink plenty of water for these to be effective.

People with sickle cell disease need extra folic acid (also known as *folate* or *vitamin B*) to produce red blood cells more quickly. This can be found in foods such as green leafy vegetables, grains and fresh fruits. You also should consult your child's doctor about whether or not to give a folic acid supplement and, if so, how much your child should take.

Doctors are also studying some other nutrients and foods that might aid people with sickle cell. These include omega fatty acids, magnesium, zinc, African yams, antioxidants, and certain herbs. Ask your doctor to keep you posted on research updates as they become available.

TEACHER—EMPLOYER GUIDE

This is a guide that can be typed in a letter for your teachers and/or employers. (This guide is on the Sickle Cell Information Center web site, http://www.emory.edu/PEDS/SICKLE/, and can be printed directly from the site.)

- Sickle cell patients may be absent because of severe pain episodes caused by the blockage of blood flow to body organs or bones. Such episodes may require treatment in a hospital setting.
- Makeup work for students should be provided to keep the student current with assignments. A hospital or home based teacher may be required if the student has prolonged complications.
- Pain episodes may be prevented by allowing the individual to keep well hydrated with water. Do not limit the person's access to water as his or her requirements are increased. This will probably require frequent bathroom breaks.
- Pain episodes may also be prevented by not allowing the individual to become over-heated or exposed to cold temperatures.

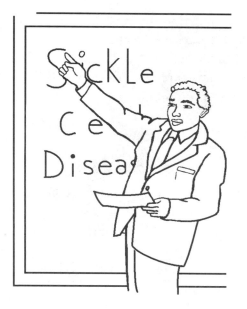

- Because of their anemia, individuals with sickle cell may tire before others and a rest period may be appropriate. Encourage gym and sports participation but let the person stop without undue attention.
- Sickle cell disease does not affect one's intelligence, but various factors of this lifelong illness may impair academic performance. These should be identified and addressed as they would be for any child. Because the life expectancy for those with sickle cell is now up in the fourth and fifth decade, academic performance is important. Those with sickle cell can become professionals as well as anyone else.
- Sickle cell patients may have a yellow tint to their eyes because of the anemia. They also may have a shorter stature and delayed puberty.
- Those with sickle cell should be treated as normally as possible with an awareness that they may have intermittent episodes of pain, infection or fatigue that can be treated and

sometimes prevented through adequate water intake, avoiding temperature extremes and over exertion.

- Learn about sickle cell and understand the challenges that may be faced. Have a plan of action with the individual to do what you can to keep him or her productive and complication free.

WHAT YOU CAN DO

- Invite a speaker from your local sickle cell foundation or clinic to educate the entire class or staff about sickle cell.
- Become involved in public awareness events, like walks, fun runs, kids' camp and fund raisers.
- Encourage blood donations and blood drives in your community. Many with sickle cell need transfusions to prevent childhood strokes and other complications.
- Support sickle cell research to provide new treatments.
- Encourage sickle cell patients to be the best they can be.

CHAPTER **6**

Sickle Cell Trait

INCIDENCE

Over 3.5 million African Americans are carriers of sickle cell trait. Sickle cell trait is the inheritance of just one sickle gene—a minute piece of genetic information that can make an enormous difference in the life one leads. Why? Because that one sickle gene, in combination with one normal gene, causes just under half the hemoglobin inside the red blood cells to be sickle hemoglobin.

One should be certain of the diagnosis because some people have been told they have sickle cell trait when they really have a variant of the disease. If in doubt, have the hemoglobin electrophoresis test repeated and read by a skilled hematologist. To make things more complicated, Hemoglobin sickle beta plus thalassemia can be misdiagnosed as sickle cell trait.

It is important to tell your health care providers that you have sickle cell trait. It is also important to understand some of the symptoms that can be seen under extreme conditions and how to avoid complications. Finally, knowing you have sickle cell trait means:

- You can pass this gene on to your future children
- Sickle cell trait will never transform into sickle cell disease

- You should have a normal life without symptoms if you avoid extremes of dehydration, low oxygen, pressure changes, or extreme exhaustion
- Certain occupations and recreational activities may cause problems
- Travel to high altitudes or deep sea diving can cause symptoms

MISDIAGNOSES

If symptoms more typical of sickle cell disease, like anemia, pains, and jaundice, are occurring, the following should be considered:

- Misdiagnosed sickle beta plus thalassemia. A person with sickle beta plus thalassemia may have symptoms of sickle cell disease. Always get tests and counsel from health care providers who understand the different types of sickle cell disease.
- Misdiagnosed sickle plus some other interacting hemoglobin like C, D, or E.
- Incorrect diagnosis. Individuals with hemoglobin SC disease are sometimes told that they have sickle trait by uninformed health professionals. This can be correctly diagnosed with a repeat hemoglobin electrophoresis.
- Sickle Cell Trait with Complications.
- Microscopic bleeding, or blood you can not see without a microscope, is the most common problem (1% to 4%) experienced by people with sickle cell trait. Bloody or cola colored urine (hematuria) is not as common. Bleeding should be evaluated by a physician who should check for other causes. Bleeding can reoccur and can be severe enough to cause anemia. Bleeding may require hospital treatment with intravenous fluids and medications to slow it down.

Individuals with bleeding into the urine should drink a lot of water before, during, and after physical exertion. Those with frequent, severe, or persistent bleeding into the urine may need to avoid activities that regularly cause episodes. Drinking a lot of water and bed rest may stop pain episodes if done quickly.

RARE COMPLICATIONS

People with sickle cell trait are generally completely normal physically and show no symptoms. Their blood evaluation is normal, with no anemia and no evidence of red cells breaking apart. There are no laboratory abnormalities other than hemoglobin AS on hemoglobin electrophoresis.

Many individuals with sickle cell trait will have a decreased ability to concentrate their urine. There may be an increased amount of urinary tract infection during pregnancy. Painless blood in the urine, or hematuria, does occur in 1% to 4% of individuals with sickle cell trait. This complication is usually not significant, but a small number of people may have difficulty with recurrent blood in the urine requiring medical intervention, transfusion, and supplemental iron therapy.

While blood in the urine of a patient with the sickle cell trait is probably not dangerous, the examining physician must be alert to the possibility that the bleeding comes from other, more serious causes, such as kidney or bladder stones, polyps, tumors, or bleeding disorders.

Complications such as splenic infarction, pain episodes, and sudden death may be caused by severe hypoxia, severe dehydration, and severe exertion.

Individuals with sickle trait have a higher risk of serious complications if they exercise at the extremes of human endurance. With extremely low oxygen and/or lack of water, complications like blood backing up in the spleen and pain episodes may occur, though rarely. (Caucasians with sickle cell trait may be at higher risk for these complications.) Drinking a lot of water regularly and building up exercise tolerance are important preventive measures.

Pain Episode. This is pain deep in the extremities, lower back, or chest. It should be treated like a sickle cell pain episode, with intravenous hydration, bed rest and pain medications.

Splenic Sequestration. The symptoms of splenic sequestration are

- abdominal pain, especially in the upper left abdominal area
- weakness, abdominal swelling, especially in the upper left abdomen.

This can happen over several minutes to hours. If you are concerned about splenic sequestration go to an emergency room and tell the medical staff that you have sickle cell trait. Splenic sequestration may not be a complication the staff is aware of if they do not see many sickle cell patients. Treatment includes blood transfusions, and potential spleen removal.

Multi-Organ Failure and Sudden Death. There have been case reports in military and sports medical journals of sudden collapse and death in individuals with sickle cell trait as a result of extreme physical activity and little hydration. In one military study of two million recruits, a 28-fold increase in unexplained exercise related deaths occurred in those with sickle cell trait, compared to similar age, sex, and race matched non sickle cell trait recruits. About half of these deaths were from heat illness and the other half had no other detectable cause except sickle cell trait.

TRAVEL PRECAUTIONS

The higher you go, the more likely you may be to develop pain or other sickle cell related problems. People with sickle cell trait may experience trouble traveling to cities with high altitudes, such as

Denver or Mexico City. Car travel in mountain terrains may also cause problems.

Travel in pressurized aircraft is fine. Unpressurized aircraft may cause problems.

PREVENTION OF COMPLICATIONS

- Don't push the limit of your physical endurance.
- Always drink plenty of water and keep a water bottle with you while exercising.
- Take rest breaks to allow the body to cool down and recover from exercise.
- Always build up slowly to a desired level of exercise.
- If traveling to a higher altitude, allow a few days to acclimate your body to the pressure and oxygen differences.
- Do not exercise immediately, but acclimate yourself to the new area. Avoid exercising in the heat of the day. It is best to walk or run in the morning or evening.

Certain sports are especially risky, for example, scuba diving, sky diving, and skiing at high elevations. Sports and occupations that cause physical exertion in the heat, pressure changes, low oxygen, or dehydration all may cause complications.

CHAPTER 7

General Medical Care

You want to be sure that you and your loved ones get the best possible medical care. You can help do this by understanding not just your disease but also the medical and non-medical teams that can help you, and the centers and agencies you can turn to for more information and support. You also need to know how best to finance the costs of care. Finally, you need to know something about the tests the doctors use to monitor your condition and the means by which they provide new treatment when necessary. In this chapter we introduce you to this information.

THE MEDICAL TEAM
DOCTORS

Doctors who help care for sickle cell patients include:

Hematologists—doctors especially trained in blood problems, including sickle cell disease. Experts in sickle cell disease usually work in sickle cell centers in a major metropolitan area.

Pediatricians—especially trained to work with children, may coordinate needed medical care.

Internists—work with adults and can coordinate care

Family practitioners — care for children *and* adults and can coordinate care.

Obstetrician-Gynecologists — care for women and manage pregnancy

Radiologists — read X-rays and scans to help diagnose problems.

Surgeons — operate on gall stones, spleens, and other conditions.

Urologists — experts in the urinary system and priapism.

Nephrologists — experts in kidney problems.

Orthopedic Surgeons — bone specialists, can operate and replace hips and shoulders damaged by avascular necrosis.

Emergency medicine specialists — staffs emergency rooms, skilled to handle emergency situations.

Anesthesia and Pain Specialists — provide pain management and anesthesia for surgery.

PA / NPS

Physician Assistants (PAs) and Nurse Practitioners (NPs) are trained to do much of what doctors do and are supervised by doctors. PAs and NPs have special training in patient education and will spend time answering questions, doing the medical checkups, seeing patients in the hospital, and coordinating care. By handling the routine care, PAs and NPs allow the sickle cell hematologist to see more patients, especially those with more critical needs.

NURSES

Nurses are teachers, medication providers, and care coordinators. They also counsel patients and family members. Nurses are the caregivers while you are in the hospital and are responsible for the twenty-four hour delivery of medications, monitoring your condition, tracking your vital signs and fluids. Nurses can be specialists, in areas such as pain management or critical care, or they can be generalists. Some nurses make home visits and can administer antibiotics and pain medication in your home.

PSYCHOLOGISTS AND PSYCHIATRISTS

Psychiatrists are medical doctors with special training in the use of medications to help depression, anxiety, and emotional disorders. Psychologists, who are not physicians, also provide counseling, testing, and emotional support for the same issues. It is important to have access to these members of the medical team when the need arises. Sickle cell is a lifelong condition that can cause emotional stresses that need professional help.

Both psychiatrists and psychologists can teach patients how to use biofeedback, distraction and relaxation techniques to help control pain. Psychologists can help determine the cause of school problems through testing and counseling.

SOCIAL WORKERS

Social workers are trained to help others solve social issues such as insurance coverage, job and school questions, housing problems, and medical disability. Social workers are experts in the local support systems and funding sources. They do crisis counseling and help families get back on their feet after setbacks. Social workers are usually employed by hospitals, sickle cell centers, and health departments. The clinic or hospital social worker should be knowledgeable about the programs available in your state.

CHAPLAINS

Chaplains are ministers employed by hospitals and clinics to help meet the spiritual needs of patients. They are available for counseling about generalized fears, fear of death, depression, and emotional stress. A healthy spiritual life is very helpful for maintaining hope and a positive outlook.

PHYSICAL THERAPISTS

Physical therapists are trained to help exercise and strengthen muscles and joints after surgery, injury, or bone infarction. They help train patients about *transcutaneous nerve stimulation* (TNS) to block chronic pain. They can help instruct patients about how to keep damaged hip and shoulder bones from getting worse.

VOCATIONAL REHABILITATION

These members of the health care team are experts in job training and retraining. They are aware of medical conditions like sickle cell and try to match patients with jobs that will not cause medical problems. If your job *is* causing you problems, this is the expert you want to see. They are usually employed by state government or by rehabilitation programs.

GENETIC COUNSELORS

Genetic counselors are trained to interpret genetic lab tests and construct special family trees called *pedigrees*. They can counsel you on the risk of having a child with genetic diseases such as sickle cell.

CLINICS

The best clinics for sickle cell patients are those whose staff is knowledgeable and compassionate. You can get recommendations from your local hematologist. You can also find out from other sickle cell patients where they get their care and if they are happy with the care. If you do not know any patients in the area, contact the nearest sickle cell association or sickle cell center for a recommendation. An updated list of clinics, sickle cell associations and centers by state is listed on the Sickle Cell Information Center at www.emory.edu/PEDS/SICKLE/clinics.htm. There is also a list of large clinics in the resource section of this book.

If you have HMO insurance, you may have an assigned caregiver and clinic. The clinician may be excellent but have very little sickle cell experience. Ask the clinician for a referral to a sickle cell expert near your home. If the clinician can't direct you, ask the clinic administrators to direct you to the best sickle cell care available in your community.

SICKLE CELL CENTERS

Sickle cell centers offer the most comprehensive services, research programs and diverse experience. These centers are usually located in large cities. It may be worth your while to visit the nearest center yearly and to have a care plan developed for your local clinic and emergency room. The best and most experienced doctors, nurses, social workers, psychologists, nurses, genetic counselors, hematologists and educators and other clinicians in the world practice at the sickle cell centers. It is worth the effort to see one of the best.

A list of the major sickle cell centers is in the reference section of this book and is continually updated on the Sickle Cell Information Center web site at www.emory.edu/PEDS/SICKLE/clinics.htm.

The sickle cell centers in New York City and Atlanta each have acute care facilities to treat pain events outside of the usual emergency room. These facilities have a success rate of 80% to 90% in getting patients better without their having to be admitted to the hospital.

EMERGENCY ROOMS

Sickle cell patients are usually dependent on their local emergency room for pain management and emergent symptoms. But help yourself before you need the emergency room. Have your regular health care provider write up an emergency room plan with your medical history, physical findings, lab values, and medications to use for pain. Have this plan placed in a notebook in your local emergency room or in your hospital chart. Keep one copy to show the nurses and physicians in the emergency room (ER) when you do go.

You must be proactive when dealing with staff in the ER. For a particular hospital, identify *before* you need them one, or several, nurse and physician champions for sickle cell patients—people who can make sure you get the proper treatment.

Free detailed sickle cell guidelines for healthcare providers are available twenty-four hours, seven days a week,on the Sickle Cell Information website at www.emory.edu/PEDS/SICKLE.

SICKLE CELL FOUNDATIONS

Many cities and communities have sickle cell foundations that provide sickle cell blood tests, and community screening at health fairs and at high schools. These foundations can provide genetic counseling, education, scholarships, summer camps, home visits, financial aid, transportation and support groups. Most do not provide medical services, but a few foundations have nurses and trained counselors on staff to provide limited medical care.

The main national organization for the various community foundations is The Sickle Cell Disease Association of America (SCDAA). Its goal is "to find a cure and improve the quality of life for those who are afflicted and their families." The SCDAA publishes and distributes, to parents and teachers, educational materials for living and coping with sickle cell disease. The contact information is listed in the reference section of this book.

Their website: www.sicklecelldisease.org has a listing by state of all of the member organizations and their contact information. The local office of SCDAA is a valuable resource of help and support. You may also wish to volunteer at the local office and become a resource yourself.

COST OF CARE

The least expensive treatment is preventive care—regular check-ups with your sickle cell provider. This is about $200 per visit.

A sickle cell patient's biggest cost is the hospital charge for in-patient stays. The average hospital stay for a sickle cell patient is five days, at a cost of $6500. Preventive measures that reduce the need to stay in the hospital will reduce costs dramatically.

The cost will vary city to city and hospital to hospital. Emergency visits to the local emergency room account for the next largest expense. These charges can be anywhere from $200 to $1000 per visit. In 1400 sickle cell patients followed at the Georgia

Comprehensive Sickle Cell Center at Grady Hospital in Atlanta, Georgia, the average number of emergency visits per year is three, and the need for admission has decreased to an average of one every two years.

Medications such as penicillin and folate are inexpensive. The preventive medication, hydroxyurea, costs about $1.25 a pill, and must be taken daily. Many drug companies have patient support programs that help you get the medication if you can't afford it. These programs usually require paperwork filled out by your doctor.

Cost for lab work and x-rays can add to the bill. The most expensive test is the MRI, which runs about $1,500.

Bone marrow transplant can cost nearly $250,000. Insurance companies must approve this procedure ahead of time.

WHAT IF I DON'T HAVE INSURANCE OR MONEY TO PAY FOR CARE?

Programs like Medicaid, available to indigent people in all states and territories of the United States, as well as Puerto Rico and Washington, D.C., can pay for practically all of your child's medical care if you qualify.

The specific requirements an individual or a family must meet to qualify for Medicaid vary from state to state. The best source of information on your state's requirements is a social worker or the local Medicaid office.

Medicaid's stated policy now is to place most subscribers into Medicaid-HMOs, but patients or their parents can apply for exemptions, which are usually granted, in the case of serious, chronic illnesses like sickle cell disease.

WHAT IF I HAVE INSURANCE BUT FIND MY OPTIONS CONFUSING?

If your employer offers healthcare insurance, arrange to talk with someone in your personnel or benefits office who can guide you to the best available options for your child and family.

If you work for a small business and no such counseling is available, seek the advice of a social worker. Many hospitals, clinics, YMCA's/YWCA's, houses of worship, and community groups offer the services of a qualified social worker free or for a nominal charge.

If no such community-based resource exists, consider hiring an independent social worker in private practice. You can find lists of social workers with phone numbers and addresses in The Yellow Pages. Friends, neighbors, doctors, nurses, and clergy are good people to ask for referrals to social workers. Usually one or two visits with a private social worker is affordable and well worth the investment.

KNOWING THE DETAILS OF YOUR HEALTH PLAN

Whatever your health plan, it pays to read it carefully and to know its regulations. If you are denied authorization for a test or treatment that your child's doctor has ordered, *be politely assertive.* You don't have to accept a "no" from the lowest ranking person on the authority ladder. If you're not satisfied with the answer you get, ask to speak to the next person up the ladder, and so on. *Polite persistence often carries the day.* This is especially true if you belong to a managed care plan or HMO.

WORKING WITH HMOS

HMO is the common term for health maintenance organization(s), also called managed care plans. Such plans assign patients to a primary care provider or PCP. This provider may be a family practitioner, a pediatrician, an internist, a gynecologist, a geriatrician (a specialist in the care of older adults), physician's assistant, or a nurse-practitioner.

The PCP is in charge of your overall care and acts as a *gatekeeper* for your medical care. That is, if you are the parent of a child with sickle cell disease, the PCP determines what tests your child will have, what treatment will be recommended, and whether a specialist should be consulted.

The guiding rule of an HMO is to keep its costs low. This means that it tends to do certain things well and other things not as well. *HMOs usually do a good job of preventive care because preventing complications saves them money.* That means they are good at making sure your child gets the proper immunizations, which is key to reducing the frequency and severity of crises. *They also, usually, do a fine job of nutritional counseling.* Good diet is important in making sure that your child grows as big and strong as the disease allows, and that the child's anemia is held in check.

But you may start to run into resistance with your HMO when it comes to treatments. Your doctor (PCP) may choose a less expensive treatment even though it might not be the most effective, have the fewest side effects, or be easiest for your child to do. In some HMOs, the PCP actually receives a yearly bonus that depends on how much money he or she has saved the company.

This means that the PCP may limit your child's access to a blood specialist (hematologist) because such consultations cost the HMO more money. In other cases, the PCP may prefer to put most of your child's care in the hands of a specialist rather than tie up his own limited office time in the care of a complicated case.

Some HMOs might not pay for more aggressive treatments for

sickle cell disease, like bone marrow transplantation. They argue that such programs are experimental, even though their usefulness in selected patients has been well established.

If you are denied treatment or service you think you should have, remember that HMOs have an appeals process. To be sure, it is stacked in favor of the bottom line, but some victories are possible.

WORKING WITH PPOS

PPOs, or preferred provider organizations, are another kind of health plan. In this type of plan you may or may not have a PCP as gatekeeper. Often, you can simply see any specialist who participates in the plan, *without* referral from a PCP.

Some PPOs will even pay a portion of the fees for visits to doctors outside their network, although you will be responsible for a larger portion of the fee than if you saw a doctor within the network.

Lately PPOs have introduced reforms that allow tests; for example, certain imaging procedures, that they previously did not support. PPO's often require prior approval for procedures, and, while their prior approval staff is usually pretty reasonable, the extra time involved may stop some doctors from ordering tests which require such approval.

WORKING WITH TRADITIONAL FEE FOR SERVICE PLANS

Traditional fee for service plans are the third major type of health plan. In this type of plan, which is becoming ever rarer and more expensive, you can see any doctor you want. After an annual deductible (which varies from one plan to another) has been met, the plan will pay the doctor 70% to 85% of the *approved amount* for the doctor's services. The approved amount is usually significantly less than the doctor's usual fees.

If your child's doctor accepts assignment, you will only be responsible for the portion of the approved amount not paid by the plan. If your child's doctor does not accept assignment, you will be expected to pay the doctor directly for your child's care. The plan will then reimburse you the usual percentage of the approved amount.

WORKING WITH MEDICARE

Your child may be able to get Medicare coverage if he or she is awarded social security disability. For a child to qualify, he or she must have worked on a job that withheld social security taxes. To qualify your child must stop working because of his or her medical condition.

SSI

Another social security program for the disabled is SSI. To be awarded SSI a person has to fulfill the same requirements as for social security disability, except that the applicant need never have worked. The financial award is usually less than what one receives with a disability award. This program does not lead to Medicare coverage.

FALLING THROUGH THE CRACKS

Some people just don't quality for any federal assistance program. A few states have begun to respond to this vacuum in Federal programs. New York, for instance, has a low cost health insurance program for children called Child Health Plus, which covers many of a child's basic healthcare needs. A social worker can tell you if a similar program exists in your state.

Many sickle cell clinics will provide care to your child, if indigent, at reduced fees or no charge. Many public and private voluntary hospitals will provide medical care, including high caliber specialty care, on a sliding fee scale. Again, a social worker can advise you.

COMMON LAB TESTS
CBC—RETIC COUNT

The most common blood test is the complete blood count or the CBC. This is actually several blood tests combined. It lets your healthcare provider know how the cells in the blood are doing. Some tests count the number of red blood cells, white blood cells and platelets. Others measure the *hematocrit*, which is the percentage volume of red blood cells over the total volume of blood. There is a measure called *the mean corpuscular volume* or MCV, that checks the average size of the red blood cells. If the red cells are larger than normal, it might mean you are low in folate or vitamin B12. If the red cells are smaller than normal, it may mean that you are low in iron, have a thalassemia, or have lead poisoning. The hemoglobin value is also reported.

Your health care provider closely monitors these blood values. Each person has his/her own normal baseline. In a person with sickle cell disease raising or lowering the blood values can cause serious complications.

The best check to see how the bone marrow factory is doing is a test that measures brand new red blood cells, called *reticulocytes*.

The white blood cell count is important to watch because it often rises when the body is under attack by viruses or bacteria.

Platelets also may increase because of the increased bone marrow production.

CHEMISTRY

Blood chemistry values important to know about in sickle cell disease are the LDH or *Lactate dehydrogenase,* an enzyme found inside red blood cells. In sickle cell patients this value is usually way above the normal because of the constant splitting of sickled red blood cells in fourteen days (hemolysis) rather than the normal one hundred twenty days. Another chemical released from the break-up of red blood cells is indirect *bilirubin,* a byproduct of hemoglobin recycling. When bilirubin levels go above 2, the white part of the eyes becomes yellow. This is not harmful and it comes and goes with the amount of red blood cells breaking apart.

The chemistry values ALT, AST, Alkaline phosphatase all indicate how the liver is doing. When the liver becomes irritated by infection or gall stones, these values rise.

Two other chemistry tests, the blood urea nitrogen, or BUN, and Creatinine indicate how the kidneys are doing. The higher these values, the less efficiently the kidneys are filtering toxins from the blood.

URINALYSIS AND URINE PROTEIN

A urinalysis consists of multiple tests on the urine that check how the kidney is doing and to see if there is blood or infection in the urinary tract. Too much protein released by the kidney into the urine is one of the first signs that the kidney has been damaged by the sickled red cells. Research is now looking for ways to prevent this damage using special blood pressure medications called *ACE inhibitors.*

FERRITIN

Ferritin is the best simple blood test measure of the iron level in the body. As patients have repeated blood transfusions, this level indicates the greater or lesser possibility of stroke and other complications. Iron does not leave the body without help; it deposits in many organs like the liver and heart causing damage. *Desferoxamine* is given as a slow infusion using a small needle under the skin to help the body remove excess iron.

HEMOGLOBIN ELECTROPHORESIS

Hemoglobin electrophoresis is the blood test that lets us know what types of hemoglobin are in the red blood cells. This and other methods of hemoglobin diagnosis are discussed in the diagnosis— detection chapter. Clinicians will do repeated checks of the hemoglobin S level with this test when one is on monthly blood transfusion therapy.

LOOKING FOR INFECTIONS

When clinicians suspect that an infection is present, they may order cultures of the urine, blood, sputum or joint fluid, to see if bacteria are growing and, if so, to identify them. Cultures usually take 24–48 hours to reveal if a bacteria is present. Because waiting for the results could be deadly, an antibiotic is commonly given *before* the test results are in to protect the patient.

Other tests for infection include blood tests that detect the presence of viruses like HIV, Hepatitis A,B,C,D,E, mononucleosis, and CMV.

COMMON PROCEDURES
IV FLUIDS

Sickle cell pain and complications can be caused by a lack of water inside the red cells. A quick way to put the water back into the red cells is by intravenous (IV) fluids. A small plastic tube is placed in a vein and water with 5% glucose(sugar) is allowed to drip into the blood stream. Drinking water can have the same re-hydrating effect, but it is difficult to drink enough water when pain is present to reduce the pain.

TRANSFUSION THERAPY

Blood transfusions are necessary when the number of blood cells becomes too low, to treat or prevent a stroke, to treat acute chest syndrome, to treat splenic sequestration, and to treat priapism. Transfusions may be given before surgery to prevent complications. In a *simple transfusion* a bag of donor red blood cells is dripped into a vein by an IV over a few hours. An *exchange transfusion* involves removing sickle blood cells from the person while transfusing in the donor red cells. This is necessary in emergent situations or when the blood count is too high and a transfusion is necessary to lower the sickle hemoglobin.

There are a number of important complications that may occur with transfusion. The most important include too much blood volume (overload), alloimmunization, iron overload, and exposure to infections. *Fluid overload* is usually caused by doing the transfusion too quickly without the body having time to adjust to the extra red cells and fluid. This can cause a stroke or a pain episode from the blood sludging (or becoming thick and slow flowing).

Alloimmunization is a common problem occurring in about one quarter of transfused sickle patients. The patient's immune system begins to see the donor blood cells as foreign and attacks them. This causes delayed transfusion reactions, and development of autoantibodies, making it difficult to find a blood donor match. Prevention of alloimmunization and delayed transfusion reactions is helped by providing a record of previous transfusions, reactions, and alloantibodies to the parent and/or patient.

Sensitized individuals should wear identification bracelets that provide alloantibody information and a number to call to obtain their transfusion history. Screening for alloantibodies six to eight weeks

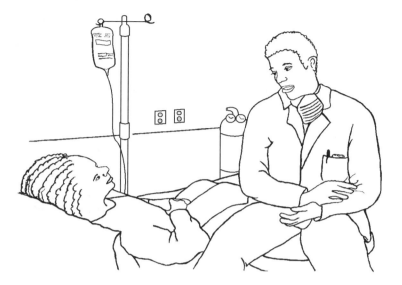

after transfusion will document new antibodies that may disappear if there is a prolonged period without transfusion, but still cause delayed transfusion reactions if further transfusions are required.

Limiting the number of units transfused is also important. The likelihood of causing antibodies can be reduced by using donors of the same ethnic background as the patient.

Iron overload can only be prevented by limiting the amount of red blood cells transfused. Exchange transfusion, where sickle blood is removed as new donor blood is transfused in, is another method of limiting iron overload.

Testing for infectious agents markedly reduces, but does not eliminate, exposure to hepatitis, AIDS, and other viral diseases. If you received transfusions from 1975 through 1985 you should be offered counseling about possible HIV infection. Others given screened blood should be tested for hepatitis or HIV on request or in clinical situations where infection is likely.

It is extremely important for all patients and parents to carry records of all their transfusions, reactions, and alloantibodies. These should be presented to any new physician and to those giving transfusions. A running total of units transfused will help track the iron put in your body.

BLOOD THICKNESS AND TISSUE OXYGENATION

Whole blood thickness (viscosity) and its ability to flow quickly is often increased during complications in sickle cell disease. Transfusions are needed during certain complications because oxygen carrying is increased and the red blood cells containing sickle hemoglobin are diluted by cells with normal hemoglobin. Regular transfusions prevent strokes. Transfusions may be lifesaving during aplastic and sequestration crises.

Special considerations to be aware of when getting a transfusion are:

- exposure to infections
- iron overload
- too much fluid that may make blood flow slow too much
- exposure to anti-bodies, which makes it difficult to find matching blood.

CHELATION THERAPY FOR IRON REMOVAL

The human body does not get rid of iron well. Iron overload occurs in people with sickle cell syndromes who have had many red cell transfusions. The body's iron stores become full after receiving approximately 20-30 transfusions. More iron accumulation beyond this point leads to problems in the heart, liver, and endocrine organs. All endocrine glands can be affected, but most commonly the pancreas (leading to diabetes mellitus), anterior pituitary (causing short stature), parathyroid (causing low calcium), and thyroid.

The blood test Serum ferritin is the most frequently used measure of total body iron. Hepatic iron concentration (HIC) is considered to be the most accurate measure of total body iron. This test involves analyzing a sample of the liver and is done by a specialist.

Deferoxamine mesylate (Desferrioxamine, Desferal, DF) is the only iron remover or chelator approved for use in the United States. Iron bound to DF is excreted in the urine and turns the urine pink. DF is only effective for chronic chelation therapy when given through a needle under the skin. DF has been in regular use for treatment of transfusional iron overload since the mid-1970s. It is most frequently given as a subcutaneous infusion over 8-12 hours at least five nights a week using a small pump.

Initiation of deferoxamine therapy should be considered if *any* of the following occur:

- After 20-25 transfusions
- Transferrin saturation (Fe/TIBC ratio) is greater than 80%
- Ferritin level is 2000 or higher
- Hepatic iron concentration is greater than 3 mg/gm of dry weight

Before starting DF therapy, tests of hearing, vision, heart function, liver function, kidney function, and growth and development are recommended.

Annual reassessment of these parameters, as well as calcium metabolism, and endocrine function is suggested.

ULTRASOUND

Ultrasound painlessly uses sound waves to bounce back images of body organs. It can detect gall stones, spleen size, and if a baby is doing well in the mother's womb.

PULMONARY FUNCTION TESTS

Pulmonary function tests are breathing tests to see how much air the lungs are moving in and out. In sickle cell disease it's important that the lungs work well because anything that interferes with oxygen getting to the red blood cells will increase the sickling inside the body.

EYE EXAMINATIONS

Sickle cell disease, especially type SC, can cause damage to the blood vessels in the back of the eye. The signs of early blood vessel damage can be seen by eye doctors, and treatment using lasers can prevent future damage. *We recommend that all sickle cell patients have a complete eye examination once a year to check for this early damage.*

HEARING TESTS

Sickle cell disease can cause damage to the nerves involved in hearing. Annual hearing tests are important to detect hearing loss and prevent school and work problems.

TCD

Transcranial Doppler or TCD is another painless ultrasound test that measures the speed and turbulence of blood flowing through the large blood vessels supplying the brain. When a blood cell is about to close over because of sickle cell damage, it works a little like blocking the end of a running hose with your finger—the water comes out faster, with increased sound. The TCD is the best, non-painful way to predict which children are at risk for having a stroke. Such cases can be treated with preventive blood transfusion therapy.

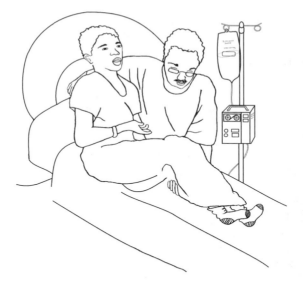

CT AND MRI SCAN

A Computerized Tomography (CT) scan is a special x-ray that allows a cross sectional view of the organs in the body. It can detect the presence of stroke, blood, tumors, growths, swelling, and blockages within the body. Magnetic Resonance Imaging (MRI) uses a large powerful magnet to make pictures of the internal organs and blood vessels.

X-RAYS

The clinicians may order x-rays of the chest when looking for pneumonia, or chest syndrome. Bone x-rays may help diagnose damage due to sickle cells or infection. This is still the most cost-effective way to look for certain complications.

BONE SCANS

Sometimes clinicians cannot tell if an infection is present in the bones. A substance that "lights-up" in areas of infection is given by

IV and the scanner traces where the substance goes. If it concentrates in one area of bone, an infection is likely and special treatment can be given.

PORTS FOR IV ACCESS

Sickle cell patients get a lot of IVs and blood tests done over the years, causing the veins to be hard and not usable. When the health care providers must search and stick multiple places just to get blood samples and give medications and fluids, it may be time to consider a port. Ports are plastic catheters put into a large vein in the arm or chest with a small round quarter sized chamber put under the skin. This chamber has a special self sealing top that can be punctured multiple times by special bent huber needles. The port gives health care providers a quick and reliable access to get blood samples and give IV fluids, blood and medications.

The good news is that with the help of such ports you have close to a sure thing, requiring one needle stick. The bad news is that these ports do not last forever and must be replaced. They can become clotted and infected if improperly cleaned and handled. The port must be flushed with a weak heparin solution once a month to prevent blood from clotting within the tubing. The port must be accessed using a sterile technique to keep bacteria from getting into the port and your blood stream. It is good for you to learn all about the sterile technique and the correct needles to use to prevent health care providers who are not familiar with ports from causing an infection.

IN THE HOSPITAL

If you or a family member needs to be admitted to the hospital, there are some matters that could make the stay more comfortable. If pain is a major issue, ask for a PCA (patient controlled analgesia pump), which gives you some control over the timing and dosage

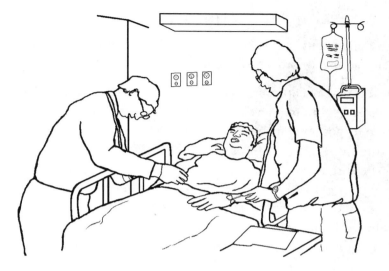

of pain medication. If PCA is not an option, ask your doctor to use long acting pain medications such as MS Contin™ or Oxycontin™.

Whenever you are in bed for more than a day you should use an incentive spirometer or blow bottle. This device exercises the lungs and prevents acute chest syndrome.

Be a teacher. Many nurses and other health care providers have not cared for a lot of sickle cell patients. Do some gentle teaching about the disease and its impact on your life. This will help build empathy in the workers.

Keep track of fluids you drink, those you get from IV, and track how much urine you excrete. The IV fluid of choice is D5W or sugar water. This fluid forces water into the dehydrated red blood cells and may reverse the sickling.

Get out of bed and walk as much as possible if you are able and allowed to do so.

Be sure to ask questions about what is going on, including your tests and the results.

SURGERY

If you or a family member is scheduled for surgery, here is what you need to know in order make the experience as safe as possible.

- You may need to have a simple blood transfusion to get your hemoglobin to a level of 10. Studies have shown that this prevents post-operative complications such as acute chest syndrome. The transfusion should be given a week or two before the surgery.
- If your hemoglobin is already 10 or higher, your doctor may want to do an exchange transfusion to keep from making your blood sludge, clot, and cause complications.
- Tell the anesthesiologist (the doctor who puts you to sleep for the surgery) that you have sickle cell disease. It is important that you are kept warm, well hydrated, and well oxygenated before, during, and after the surgery to prevent a pain episode.
- You should be placed on an incentive spirometer or blow bottle to exercise your lungs after the surgery. This will help prevent acute chest syndrome.

INFORMATION TO KEEP

You should keep a mini-medical record of all of the important complications you have had, your medication allergies, your usual lab values, the pain medications that normally work for you, and your doctor's name and phone number. It is especially important to carry this information when you travel away from home, where you may have to visit a new hospital. A sample of critical information you should carry with you at all times is in the resources chapter.

PART TWO

DEVELOPMENTAL ISSUES

CHAPTER **8**

Sickle Cell Disease: Birth to Six Years

T he symptoms of sickle cell disease, and its treatment, change over the course of the patient's life. In the next chapters we will talk about these stages of development, beginning with infancy and early childhood.

Let's start with what parents and health providers want to keep focussed on. First, the clinical issues, period by period.

CLINICAL ISSUES
BIRTH TO 6 MONTHS

- Find a sickle cell clinic or see a physician with sickle cell experience.
- Learn all you can about sickle cell disease symptoms and prevention.
- Schedule physician clinic examinations once a month, usually when immunizations are due.
- Begin giving the child penicillin, 125 mg liquid by mouth twice a day, by two months of age.
- Learn how to recognize fever, how to take temperature, and the importance of penicillin.

- Have the child's hemoglobin electrophoresis repeated to confirm the sickle cell diagnosis.
- Get appropriate immunizations, especially the pneumococcal vaccine Prevnar™.
- If you are grieving about your child having sickle cell disease, share that grief with friends, ministers, or counselors.

6 MONTHS TO 1 YEAR

- Begin giving the child folic acid, 1 mg.
- Learn about nutrition, prevention of complications and accidents, hand-foot syndrome, recognizing illness, and spleen sequestration.
- Schedule clinic visits for every two months.
- Continue all immunizations.
- Have your extended family tested for sickle cell and a family pedigree made.
- Meet with a genetic counselor.

1 TO 2 YEARS

- Continue all immunizations.
- Discuss with your doctor pain control, growth /development, and issues related to lifelong disease.
- Schedule clinic visits every 3 months.
- Each clinic visit should include a physical examination, CBC and reticulocyte count.
- Get the pneumococcal vaccine, 23 valent, at age 2.
- Blood chemistries should be done twice a year.
- Watch for signs of infection, stroke, and increasing anemia.
- Learn the importance of hydration and diet.

2 TO 6 YEARS

- Increase the penicillin dose to 250 mg twice a day, by mouth, and continue folic acid.
- Learn about normal growth and development milestones, hydration, avoidance of over-dependence, setting limits.
- Schedule clinic visits every 3 months.
- Complete all immunizations.
- Learn about pain management principles.
- Educate school nurses/teachers about sickle cell with handouts, meetings, and letters.

PSYCHO-SOCIAL ISSUES

During this period a child goes through many miraculous changes. She'll take her first step, begin to talk, and develop a growing sense of herself as a social being. For the parents of children with sickle cell disease, these changes bring their own problems. During this period your child will become aware that her physical life is different from her companions'. It is not easy to tell a child she has an illness she may have to carry with her for a lifetime. Nor is it easy to cope with a child who is simply fed up with the demands of chronic disease, and sometimes refuses to cooperate.

TALKING WITH YOUR CHILD

Talking with a child about chronic disease should take place only in stages, according to the child's level of understanding at the time. Of course your child will have questions. So will your other children. The best policy, is to answer your children's questions simply, factually, in terms they can understand. Don't be grim or sad, but don't lie or sugar-coat the truth either. Kids will always see through our lies, however well-intentioned, and a certain amount of precious trust will be lost.

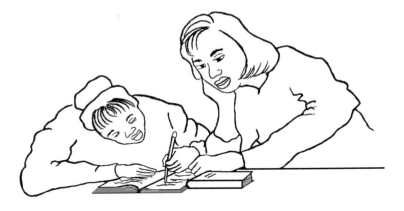

WHAT TO DO WHEN YOUR CHILD ACTS OUT

Like anyone with a chronic disease, your child will sometimes get fedup with taking pills, seeing doctors, and going for blood tests. A child's resistance to treatment can be heart breaking. It peaks in the preteen and teen years, when some kids not only won't cooperate but deliberately do things that they know can provoke sickle cell crises—like not drinking enough water—in order to manipulate the rest of the family.

At an early age children learn that when they have a pain episode they get a lot of extra attention and, more often than not, get their way. Sometimes, if they get desperate, they may resist treatment, feeling that such resistance gives them power.

The best way to avoid these attention and power seeking episodes is to keep the lines of communication with your child open. If you can do that, your child, should he choose to act out, can usually be talked back into good sense. But sometimes even a parent's best efforts may fail. That's when family counseling may be helpful.

In general, what the child, or any person suffering a disability, wants to know is what to expect from the disease, and what to expect from the health care system in the way of treatment. The better the child is prepared for the pain and discomfort that the disease, and sometimes the treatment itself, may bring, the better he or she will be able to go along with it.

Your own patience and love will make itself felt. Trust that. In the bad times, friends, relatives, and counselors can help. So can support groups. Be willing to lean on those who will gladly help you carry the weight.

COMMON MANIFESTATIONS

Knowing what symptoms to expect prepares you to react to them. Here are signs to watch for as your child grows.

NEWBORN—2 MONTHS OLD

Babies of this age generally have no symptoms of sickle cell disease because they still have enough fetal blood to protect them against the effects of sickle hemoglobin or hemoglobin S.

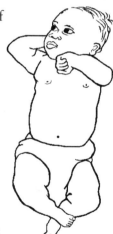

THREE MONTHS— 6 MONTHS OLD

Symptoms of sickle cell disease often start at this age, when the baby's fetal hemoglobin is quickly being replaced by adult sickle hemoglobin. The first warning sign in the child is often a painful swelling of its fingers and toes, referred to as *hand-foot syndrome,* or *acute sickle dactylitis.* This is the result of an imbalance between the demand for, and the supply of, blood in these fingers and toes. Rapidly growing bone marrow chokes off its own blood supply by narrowing, or compressing, the blood vessels.

Often there is accompanying fever because of associated infections. If there is a family history of sickle cell disease or trait, parents and other caregivers should check with their doctors about sickle cell anemia when infants have their first episode of fever. In a baby with sickle cell disease, fever can be caused by a life-threatening infection.

Signs of fever in the baby include:

- extreme crankiness
- incessant crying
- rapid breathing
- screaming even when touched or held by family members
- lack of energy
- poor appetite
- decrease in the number of wet diapers (which indicates dehydration)

In the United States and other parts of the world where malaria has been eliminated, the first episode of sickle cell pain is often brought on by bacterial infection. Where malaria is still common, the first episode is typically brought on by malarial infection.

SIX MONTHS—5 YEARS

For the sickle cell patient this period of childhood is characterized by

- a progressive breakdown of the child's red blood cells and subsequent anemia that shows itself in pallor (paleness) of the palms, soles, lips, and eyelids
- jaundice, or yellow discoloration of the skin and the whites of the eyes due to the deposition of bilirubin, a pigment generated from the breakdown of hemoglobin

COMPLICATIONS

Unfortunately, sickle cell disease can cause any number of secondary complications. Being familiar with them prepares you to cope with them should they develop.

HAND-FOOT SYNDROME

Sickle dactylitis, or hand-foot syndrome, is one of the first complications seen in sickle cell disease, usually occurring between ages six months and two years. One third to one half of patients may experience this complication during early childhood; it is very rare in later life.

Hand-foot syndrome is the result of blocked blood flow and damage to the small bones of the fingers and toes, which causes a rapid, painful expansion of the bone marrow cavity of these small bones. This painful swelling of the back of both hands and feet was the symptom that led to diagnosis before newborn screening became common.

Treatment of hand-foot syndrome includes hydration and pain control with acetaminophen. Bone changes occurring during episodes of dactylitis can be caused by, or mistaken for, osteomyelitis (infection in the bone).

FEVER AND INFECTIONS

Bacterial infections are the most common cause of death in children with sickle cell disease during the first five years of life. Those under three years are at greatest risk for life threatening infections, but dangerous infections can be seen at any age. The sickle cell patient's decreased ability to fight off overwhelming infection is the result of the spleen not working properly. The spleen is the body's major defense against deadly germs. Serious infections such as blood infections (sepsis), infection surrounding the brain (meningitis), and lung infection (pneumonia) caused by these germs are common and often may be life-threatening.

The bones and joints may also become infected. Infections of the bladder and kidney are more common and may be more severe than in individuals without sickle cell disease. Lives can be saved by detecting these infections early and treating them with the proper antibiotic.

Preventive measures include:

- giving daily penicillin at birth until age six
- giving pneumococcal conjugate and hemophilus b vaccines, immunization for hepatitis, meningococcus, and influenza, and routine immunization for childhood diseases
- Washing hands after bathroom breaks
- not eating undercooked meat, which can contain germs that can enter the blood from the digestive system
- knowing how to check for fever and learning what to do about it.

All sickle cell patients with a fever should consider it a a top emergency, and consult a doctor immediately.

SPLENIC SEQUESTRATION

The spleen is an organ in the upper-left area of the abdomen, under the lower ribs. The spleen filters out abnormal red blood cells and helps the body's immune system fight infection. Sometimes, as in the case of sickle cell disease, red blood cells can be trapped in the spleen, a condition known as splenic sequestration. This is similar to bleeding internally because the blood trapped in the spleen cannot circulate to the heart or brain. This condition can range from mild to life-threatening, depending on how much of the body's red blood cells are trapped.

Splenic sequestration is characterized by a sudden pooling of unusually large amounts of blood in the spleen, which enlarges rapidly as a result. The movement of blood from general circulation into the spleen can lead to shock or circulatory collapse.

Patients experiencing this episode may show any signs of these:

- rapid heartbeat (tachycardia)
- shortness of breath
- dizziness
- tiredness and weakness
- stomach swelling—left upper area (due to the enlarging spleen)
- fever

Doctors detect splenic sequestration by feeling for the enlarged spleen and testing for low red-blood cell counts. You can learn how to feel for an enlarged spleen. It only takes some training and practice. Your health care provider can teach this to you when you bring in your child for a checkup.

The use of a wooden tongue depressor as a "spleen measuring stick" provides an accurate way of assessing and recording spleen size at home and in the clinic. In small children, one end can be placed on the left nipple and the distance to the spleen tip recorded in ink and dated. In older children, the distance from the ribs to the spleen tip in the left nipple line is recorded. Limits can be set by drawing red lines in ink and instructing the parent to being the child for immediate care if the spleen is increased to the line. Parents should check the spleen size on a regular basis and whenever the child appears ill. Names and phone numbers of people who need to be contacted can be written on the back of the spleen stick. Parents should bring the spleen stick with them to every follow-up and emergency visit.

If your child is doing well, then just feel for the spleen several times a week just to get practice. You should always feel for an enlarged spleen if your child:

- looks pale, which may be a sign of blood loss. In darker-skinned people, paleness may be easier to detect by looking at the lips, the inner eyelids, and the fingernail beds. Usually these areas are red or dark pink, but if they look light pink or white, then the child is pale.
- seems unusually tired, another sign of a low blood count
- is unusually cranky or irritable, and perhaps has a headache. When the red blood cell count is very low, oxygen delivery to the brain may be inadequate, causing a headache
- is sensitive to touch in the upper-left part of the abdomen—the area overlying the spleen.

If you suspect that your child has an enlarged spleen or if she is displaying any of the above symptoms, take her immediately for a medical evaluation. In a child with sickle cell disease, splenic sequestration can be extremely serious, and speedy evaluation and treatment may save her life.

Splenic sequestration may happen more than once. To prevent this, your doctor may start you on a monthly blood transfusion program or schedule surgery to remove the spleen, a procedure known as an elective splenectomy.

STROKES:
BLOCKED BLOOD FLOW TO THE BRAIN

Strokes are common in children with sickle syndromes. Strokes may occur in the first year of life and 80% occur before the age of twenty. There is a very high recurrence rate, approaching 85% in the three years after the first episode. Symptoms of a new or impending stroke include:

- seizures
- slurred speech
- fainting

- weakness and loss of sensation (numb feeling in the face, arms, or legs)

Stroke occurs when blood flow is blocked to a part of the brain by sickled cells or by bleeding from a burst blood vessel. Stroke is an emergency problem requiring hospital admission, MRI or CT scans, and immediate blood transfusions. Special rehabilitation may be needed with physical and speech therapy to recover skills that may have been damaged.

More commonly, smaller strokes may cause subtle changes in the child's personality or thinking and may leave temporary or permanent function problems. In some strokes, the vessels supplying the brain are blocked for only a short time; this is called a *transient ischemic attack* or TIA. A TIA is a serious warning signal to start preventive strategies with monthly blood transfusions. This monthly treatment keeps the hemoglobin S level at less than 30%. This helps prevent the first major stroke and can help prevent future strokes if one has occurred.

You cannot stop monthly transfusions once they've started, because stopping them would make a stroke likely to occur. And remember: monthly blood transfusions cause iron overload. They mean exposure to other people's blood, which can build up to a reaction, and it also means exposure to infectious diseases.

Bone marrow transplantation from an HLA matched brother or sister may offer children who have had strokes the best chance for a more normal life. Children with increased risk for stroke may be detected by Transcranial Doppler (TCD) Ultrasound screening (see next section).

Although "clot busters" are often used in vasoocclusive stroke that is not associated with sickle cell disease, their role in early treatment of strokes in those with sickle cell disease has not yet been tested.

In general, the medical team treats stroke victims by:

- supporting breathing and heart functions
- preventing bedsores
- preventing aspiration of food
- supporting good nutrition
- avoiding infection
- aggressively using physical and occupational therapy to prevent loss of joint flexibility and muscle strength and other rehabilitation for speech, memory, or other issues.

TCD AND STROKE PREVENTION

Sickle cell disease is one of the few conditions associated with childhood stroke, and occurs in 8% to 12% of children with certain types of sickle cell disease: HbSS and HbS beta-zero thalassemia. Stroke in these children usually results from a narrowing or closure of arteries supplying blood flow to the brain. Transcranial Doppler ultrasound (TCD) is a device that uses painless sound waves to detect areas of increased blood flow in the blood vessels of the brain. When the blood vessels are narrowed due to sickle cell damage, the blood makes a louder noise as it travels faster through the narrow area. This is like the noise in a water hose when you make the hose bend. When this test detects a constriction, or narrowing, of the blood vessels, there is a greater risk of having a stroke and further testing is necessary.

Studies have shown that transfusions did markedly reduce the risk of the first stroke in high risk children with positive TCD results. Annual TCD screening is recommended for all children with sickle cell disease type Hb SS and S beta 0 Thal between the ages of two and sixteen. A listing of centers with approved TCD screening capability can be found on the Sickle Cell Information Center website.

ACUTE CHEST PAIN

Children with sickle cell disease may experience chest pain as a result of

- blocked blood flow to the lungs
- infection
- pneumonia
- part of the "all over" pain of a pain episode.

Acute Chest Syndrome occurs when there is blocked blood flow to the lungs from infection. The person may have chest pain when they breath in and out, fever, weakness, or a high white blood cell count. This medical emergency is a common cause of hospitalization.

PAIN EVENTS

Pain episode is the most frequent acute symptom of sickle cell disease. While some patients may go for years without an episode, others may have an episode once or twice a year. Some of these may be very severe, requiring narcotic painkillers and intravenous fluids.

While some pain crises may occur without an obvious trigger factor, the triggers for most pain crises are:

- fever
- low oxygen levels
- *acidosis* (a change in the blood chemistry to the acidic side caused by infection, exhaustion, drug reactions, liver, kidney, or lung problems)
- stress
- chilly temperatures
- dehydration

These triggers can all lead to sickling of the red blood cells with clumping of groups of sickled cells and blockage of blood vessels. The resulting low blood flow to the target tissue causes pain.

Pain crises often involve the arms and legs, as well as the head, abdomen, chest, and back, depending upon which blood vessel is being blocked. The pain episode may be extensive, causing severe bone pain and secondary infection of the bone and bone marrow.

Pain episode is commonly treated with liberal amounts of oral and/or intravenous fluids, oral or injectable pain medicines, and treatment of the triggers that caused the pain.

Abdominal organs may be affected during a pain crises. Repeated damage to the spleen eventually leads to its destruction through a condition called *auto-splenectomy*. The loss of the spleen can in turn increase a person's risk for serious infections. This happens early in life for those with Hb SS and later in life for those with Hb SC or Hb S beta Thalassemia.

Other abdominal organs besides the spleen may be affected during pain crises, and the symptoms may resemble the symptoms of appendicitis or gall bladder attacks. In fact, abdominal pain episode and an abdominal surgical emergency can sometimes happen at the same time.

MORE SEVERE ANEMIA

In sickle cell patients, anemia, or a less than normal number of red blood cells, is lifelong, starting in the first year of life as the fetal hemoglobin level falls. The average red blood cell life span is reduced from a normal 120 days to an average of ten to twenty days. This causes the bone marrow factory to work overtime in order to make new red blood cells at a faster rate. When red blood cells break apart, the hemoglobin inside is converted to bilirubin, which can make the white part of the eyes look yellow, or jaundice. In later childhood and early adult life, the excess bilirubin causes gall-stones.

Splenic sequestration episode occurs when the sickled red blood cells become trapped in the small blood vessels inside the spleen. This is a cause of anemia (discussed in detail in the Sequestration section).

When the bone marrow factory stops making new red blood cells, it is called an *aplastic episode*. It occurs most commonly during early childhood, but it can occur at any age. The person with this episode has all of the symptoms of having fewer red blood cells, including increasing tiredness, weakness, shortness of breath, dizziness upon standing, and increasing paleness.

Treatment of an aplastic episode starts with a careful decision about whether to give a blood transfusion. (Too rapid a correction of the low hemoglobin can lead to fluid overload and congestive heart failure.) If the cause of the infection is bacterial, antibiotic therapy may be indicated as well.

As we explained earlier, those with sickle cell diseases already have a shortened red blood cell life span as the result of the speeded-up destruction of the rigid red blood cells by the body's filter system. When there is an additional genetic red blood cell problem, and especially when infection is present, red blood cell destruction (hemolysis) is further accelerated.

Treatment for a hemolytic episode is with blood transfusion, fluids, and treatment of any infection.

PREVENTIVE MEASURES
PENICILLIN

Because infections are among the greatest dangers to those with sickle cell disease, all children from birth until age six should be given daily penicillin. The low dose of penicillin is not enough antibiotic to rid the body of an invading infection, but it helps the body to defend itself until you can get the child to a medical facility for more powerful antibiotics. The usual penicillin dose for newborns until age two is 125 mg twice a day as a liquid. At age two the dose goes up to 250 mg twice a day. This simple low dose penicillin treatment has saved many patients' lives

VACCINATION

Children with sickle cell disease should have all of the immunizations recommended for other children. Immunizations help the body build natural defenses against invading germs and viruses. The new pneumococcal poly valent vaccine named Prevnar™ is a breakthrough that gives protection from birth through the vulnerable early childhood period. Vaccination, plus daily penicillin, will reduce the chance that fatal pneumococcal infection will occur. It is not a guarantee, so parents must be on the watch for signs of infection, mainly fever.

FARMS

For general prevention remember FARMS—

F is for *Fluids and Fever.* Have your child drink plenty of water. If you detect a fever, see your health care provider right away.

A is for *Air.* Make sure you get enough oxygen, especially in unpressurized airplanes. If your child has asthma make sure he takes his medication to prevent low oxygen levels.

R is for *Rest.* Make sure your child gets plenty of sleep, does not overdo it, and takes plenty of breaks when his body feels tired.

M is for *Prevention Medications,* like daily penicillin for children under six or hydrea for pain prevention. The vitamin folate is needed to make new red blood cells.

S is for *Situations* to avoid, like getting too hot or cold, avoiding exercise, working or playing outdoors without the proper clothing for the season, getting dehydrated, and not taking adequate rest and hydration breaks. Remember to

- carry a water bottle with you and keep drinking.
- avoid swimming pools that are too cold or hot tubs that are too hot.
- avoid emotional stress by pacing projects and work.
- avoid situations that you know are upsetting.

INCENTIVE SPIROMETERS

Incentive spirometers, or blow bottles, should be used by the child during any pain episode or event that causes bed rest. The blow bottle is a way to keep the lung's air sacks open and allow oxygen to get to the red blood cells. Using the blow bottle can help prevent deadly chest syndrome.

BONE MARROW TRANSPLANT

Bone marrow transplantation may be considered if there are dangerous complications like stroke and acute chest syndrome or frequent pain episodes. The child needs to have a HLA matched donor from a brother or sister. Successful bone marrow transplant has cured several children worldwide from having sickle cell disease. The procedure has a risk of death in up to 8% of those going through it. The procedure takes several months and costs nearly $250,000. A full description of bone marrow transplant is in the chapter on new treatment and research.

Table 5

Sickle Immunization Schedule adapted from the AAP 2001 recommendations

Birth or First visit	**Hepatitis B vaccine #1**
1 Month	Hepatitis B vaccine #2 (or 4 weeks after #1)
2 Months	DTaP, IPV, Hib, PCV7
4 Months	DTaP, IPV, Hib, PCV7
6 Months	DTaP, Hib, PCV7, Hepatitis B vaccine #3 (or 6 months after #2)
7 to 11 Months	Hib two doses 2 months apart
12 Months	PPD, Influenza*, Varicella, PCV7
12 to 14 Months	Hib one dose
15 Months	MMR Hib Booster if initial 12 -15 months
18 Months	DTaP, IPV
24 Months	Pneumovax
4 to 6 Years	DT, IPV, PPD
5 Years	Pneumovax or Booster Pneumovax
12 to 16 Years	Td, PPD, MMR booster
16 Years	Every Year Influenza*, PPD
Every 10 Years—	Td

* Sickle cell at high risk for influenza. See annual recommendations in Morbidity and Mortality Weekly Report . For details and contraindications see package inserts or

recommendations of the American Academy of Pediatrics or National Immunization Program. www.cdc.gov/nip

DTaP = Diphtheria, acellular Pertussis vaccine, Tetanus toxoid
Hib = Haemophilus B Conjugate vaccine
PPD = Tuberculin test
IPV = Inactivated Polio Vaccine
MMR = Measles, Mumps, Rubella
Pneumovax = 23 valent pneumococcal vaccine only given once if first dose after age five
PCV7 = Heptavalant conjugate pneumococcal vaccine
Td = Tetanus, Diphtheria—Adult dosage

Vaccination, penicillin prophylaxis and prompt attention to fever can prevent serious pneumococcal infections. Conjugate vaccine against S. pneumonia for infants is available—Prevnar- and should be given according to the recommended schedule along with pneumovax (see health care maintenance). Adults should receive S. pneumoniae immunization with polysaccharide vaccine once every five years and yearly influenza immunization. S.B.E. prophylaxis should be given if heart murmurs may be caused by valve pathology or if hip or other prostheses are in place.

Heptavalent Pneumococcal Conjugated Vaccine (PCV7) in children with SCD schedule up to the age of 5 years (adapted from the AAP recommendations 2000)

Age of first PCV7 dose	PCV7 Primary Series	PCV7 Booster Dose	Pneumovax
2 to 6 months	3 doses 6-8 weeks apart	1 dose 12 months	2 doses 2 years* & 5 years
7 to 11 months	3 doses 6-8 weeks apart	1 dose 24 months	2 doses 2 years* & 5 years
12 to 23 months	3 doses 6-8 weeks apart	1 dose 24 months*	2 doses 2 years* & 5 years
24 months to 4 years, no pneumovax	2 doses 6-8 weeks apart	none	2 doses 2 years* & 5 years
24 months to 4 years, had pneumovax	2 doses 6-8 weeks apart	none 5 years*	1 dose

* 6-8 weeks after last PCV7

Suggested Heptavalent Pneumococcal Conjugated Vaccine (PCV7) in children with SCD schedule 5 years and older

Age of first PCV7 dose	PCV7 Primary Series	PCV7 Booster Dose	Pneumovax
5 years & older no pneumovax	1 dose	none	1 dose*
5 years & older had pneumovax	1 dose*	none	

* 6-8 weeks after last PCV7
Some authorities recommend revaccination every 5 years with pneumovax patients at risk, practice varies among sickle cell clinics.

CHAPTER 9

6 to 12 Years

By age six the routines and procedures described in the previous chapter will be established. But some new symptoms will appear and some of the old ones will become more pronounced. You will have new tasks to do, such as monitoring your child's medical condition and helping your child keep up good preventive practices.

Also during this period, your child will start school, and you will want to have a clear understanding with his teachers and other school staff about the special requirements your child may have.

In this chapter we will talk about these new issues.

CLINICAL ISSUES

- Talk with your child's doctor about stopping penicillin.
- Schedule clinic visits every 4 to 6 months.
- Start scheduling full eye examinations every year.
- Identify Gall stones with an ultrasound test.
- Have your child screened for hearing loss and pulmonary function (breathing).

PSYCHO-SOCIAL AND PARENTING ISSUES

- Stress academic achievement, prevention of complications, and health maintenance
- Begin sex education
- Keep track of your child's psycho-social development
- Be prepared for delayed puberty
- Set limits for behavior
- Encourage good school performance
- Be sure you and your child keep doctors' appointments
- Do not let sickle cell rule the house
- Spend quality time together doing fun and memorable activities
- Allow normal activities, keeping in mind FARMS prevention.
- Try not to favor the child with sickle cell disease over other brothers and sisters, giving all quality time. There may be episodes of hospitalization where the normal daily routine is disrupted. Let the other children know what is going on and let them be involved as much as possible.

"SICK ROLE"

Give your child care and compassion when the child is well and pain free, with equal amounts for all of your children. Show this same care and compassion when the child is ill and in pain, but without making a big fuss. Avoid "rewarding" the child in times of pain and illness. Some children, and adults, who are rewarded with attention only when they are ill or in pain develop a "sick role," using pain in order to gain attention. Your aim should be to motivate the child to get better and to continue with the daily routines of school, friends, and activities.

CAMP

Many sickle cell foundations and clinics spon-
sor a sickle cell camp during the summer for
children six to twelve years old. These camps
allow the children to have fun with other
kids with sickle cell disease in a medically
supervised environment. These
camps usually have adult sickle cell
patients as counselors to help mentor the younger patients.

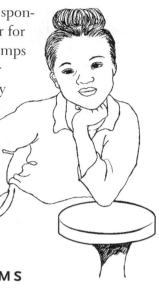

Check with the sickle cell
community group and clinic near
you to see if a camp is offered.

AGE-SPECIFIC SYMPTOMS

- The inability to concentrate urine will become more
  obvious. Affected children will urinate more often and persistent bed wetting (*enuresis*) may occur. These problems under-
  standably lead to difficulties in the child's socialization.
  Normal activities like camp, sleepovers, school trips, and even
  sitting through classes become potentially embarrassing for
  the child. Bed wetting may become a source of conflict
  between the parent and the child if the parents do not understand the cause.
- Prolonged anemia will develop. This is caused by early red
  blood cell breakdown (hemolysis). This breakdown releases
  hemoglobin into the blood stream where it is converted to
  bilirubin. Bilirubin causes the white part of the eye to turn
  yellow (jaundice).
- An enlarged spleen may be regarded as a filter for broken red
  blood cells. The spleen's job is to help get rid of them. In an
  attempt to fulfill this function in those with sickle cell disease,

the spleen enlarges. Occasionally, this organ experiences pooling of large volumes of blood; this is called a *sequestration episode*. These two processes combine to produce enlargement of the spleen.

- Your child will have an increased need for calories and energy to build new red blood cells and damaged tissue.
- Abnormal development of the jaw and/or breast bone occurs in some individuals. The bone marrow expands as it tries to accommodate the need for increased red blood cell production. The primary expansion sites include the jaws and the breast bone. Prominence of the forehead (known as *frontal bossing*), and protrusion of the jaw (known as *prognathism*) are among the abnormal bony symptoms of some people with sickle cell disease. Because the jaw protrudes, dental abnormalities and gum disease may occur more often in these children.

COMPLICATIONS

New secondary problems can develop in children with sickle cell disease during this period.

GALLSTONES

Gallstones can form in the gall bladder, which holds bile, a substance made from bilirubin, the by-product of hemoglobin recycling. Bile helps your body digest fatty foods. Because of the increased red cell hemolysis in sickle cell disease, bilirubin production is increased and this causes gallstones to form in the gall bladder.

Gall stones can cause the gall bladder to become plugged and swollen. This causes pain in the upper right area of the stomach, nausea, and vomiting. These symptoms can happen especially after eating fatty or fried foods.

If neccessary, the gall bladder can be surgically removed.

DELAYED GROWTH

Children with sickle cell may weigh less than others of the same age, though this varies from child to child. Older children and adolescents with sickle cell disease, on the average, are shorter than their peers, but this difference disappears in adulthood. Puberty may come later in both males and females with sickle cell disease. Factors contributing to the delay include the low red blood cell count, and the type of sickle cell disease.

Treatment for delayed growth includes good general nutrition, vitamins, increased calories and, on the psychological side, reassurance that normal maturation will occur.

PRIAPISM

Priapism is the painful erection of the penis caused by sickling red blood cells blocking blood flow out of the penis. Priapism usually occurs between the ages of five to thirty-five. It often occurs as a severe long episode requiring hospitalization and follows multiple episodes of short duration, termed "stuttering." Episodes may come from infection, having sexual intercourse, masturbation, or normal night-time erections. Onset in the early morning, awakening the patient, is common.

Treatment for priapism includes pain relief, medication that opens closed blood vessels, hydration, blood transfusion, and surgery. Impotence is a long-term consequence of repeated episodes in half to one-third of the cases.

KIDNEY PROBLEMS: BED WETTING, PROTEIN

The kidney has just the right conditions—low oxygen and high acid concentration—to cause red cells to sickle. The kidney is the main filter of the blood, saving or releasing water, salts, and waste products. If early damage impairs the kidney's ability to retain water it can let too much go, even when the the body is dehydrated.

When the kidney releases too much water, children may wet the bed at night and may need frequent bathroom breaks. This is important to discuss with teachers and caregivers. To help control the bedwetting problem, use an alarm that sounds when dampness is detected. These are available at most drug stores. Encourage your child to stop drinking fluids one hour before going to bed.

Over time damage to the kidney filters can cause protein to leak into the urine. This is the first sign that more damage is occurring. A special urine test for protein, with data collected over twenty-four hours, can help predict the level of damage that may occur. There is research underway to test preventive medications that may slow this kidney damage.

PREVENTIVE MEASURES

- Again, the best strategy for prevention is FARMS, as outlined in the previous chapter.
- Be sure that when your child exercises or works outdoors, he wears the proper clothing for the season, carries a water bottle and drinks plenty of water, and takes frequent rest and water breaks.
- Your child should avoid swimming pools that are too cold or hot tubs that are too hot.
- Your child should avoid emotional stress by pacing projects and work, and by avoiding situations likely to be upsetting.
- Parents and child should belong to a support group. This will often be, according to your beliefs, a church or faith-based group that can offer spiritual and emotional support.

COMPLICATIONS
TCD AND STROKE PREVENTION

Transcranial Doppler ultrasound testing should continue annually until age sixteen for children with Hb SS and Hb S beta 0 thalassemia. See the previous chapter for further information on this test as a means of stroke prevention.

HYDREA—HYDROXYUREA

Hydroxyurea therapy for pediatric sickle cell patients is in a transition zone between "experimental therapy" and "commonly accepted therapy." The treatment has been relatively uncommon among pediatric patients, more common among teenagers, and most common among adults.

While there is much still to be learned about hydroxyurea therapy for sickle cell patients, we know this:

- Hydroxyurea treatment seems to improve pain, acute chest syndrome, priapism, and abnormal red blood cell stickiness to the blood vessel wall (endothelium).
- Hydroxyurea decreases the frequency of pain episodes, though it may not completely eliminate them.
- Small studies have shown no impact of hydroxyurea on sickle cell damage to the spleen, and perhaps no impact in avascular necrosis of bones such as the hip and shoulder joint.

New information about side effects and episode reduction benefits will come out during the next several years, but at the moment, the side effects for children on hydroxyurea appear to be the same as the effects for adult patients:

Common:

- Mild nausea or upset stomach. Most patients have this only for the first few weeks at a certain dose, then the nausea goes away. Sometimes nausea is less troublesome if the hydroxyurea is taken at bedtime.
- Suppression of blood cell production.
  Mild suppression is an intended side effect of hydroxyurea, but hydroxyurea dosing needs to be carefully adjusted and blood

cell counts monitored every two to four weeks to make sure that the suppression does not become severe. Hydroxyurea may suppress the white blood cells too much, leading to increased chances of infection; suppress platelet counts too much, leading to increased chances of bleeding; or suppress red blood cell counts too much, leading to worse anemia, with fatigue and problems for heart and lung function.

Possible:

- Thinning of hair
- Darkening of skin and nails

Rare:

- Decreased kidney or liver function
- Dizziness
- Changes in mood or thought
- Excess chances of intracranial bleeding unrelated to platelet counts

All of these effects are expected to be reversible when the hydroxyurea is stopped. Generally, the medication can then be adjusted to a lower dose.

Several potential side effects of long-term hydroxyurea therapy may be:

LEUKEMIA

Some people on hydroxyurea for other blood disorders seem to have an increased rate of developing leukemia (cancer of white blood cells). However, it is possible that sickle cell disease by itself—and not the hydroxyurea treatment—predisposed those people to leukemia. Studies in groups of sickle cell patients on hydroxyurea have not revealed increased DNA damage that would make us suspicious of leukemia development.

BIRTH DEFECTS

So far, the handful of babies born to mothers on hydroxyurea for sickle cell have not had birth defects. But worry about the possibility of birth defects leads most doctors to give hydroxyurea only when there is no possibility of conception. Males or females on hydroxyurea should abstain from sex or use excellent contraception. It is not known whether being on hydroxyurea for a number of years and then stopping before conceiving a baby will help avoid the chance of birth defects.

GROWTH AND DEVELOPMENT PROBLEMS

People have worried that hydroxyurea treatment will slow the growth or development of children with sickle cell disease. A few years of tracking several dozen children has not revealed growth and development problems so far, but longer experience is needed.

HYDROXYUREA TREATMENT IN A NUTSHELL

Hydroxyurea therapy for a child with sickle cell disease has many possible benefits, several known risks, and several potential long term side effects. The full details of the levels of these risks will not be known until there have been many more years of experience with sickle cell hydroxyurea treatment.

We strongly recommend individual discussions with your child's hematologist about the risks and benefits for your child. At Grady Hospital, we generally have two or three sessions in order to:

- review the child's medical history and present condition
- discuss individualized risks and benefits

- provide reading material on these risks and benefits
- draw a panel of baseline lab tests (blood counts, vitamin B12 and folate levels, kidney function and liver function, check for hepatitis and HIV infection, test for pregnancy)
- check a brain MRI scan for any signs of stroke or abnormal blood vessels that might increase the chances of bleeding in the head.

You need to have a doctor who will follow your child very closely for blood counts and monitor for hydroxyurea related problems and for other sickle cell problems.

ALTERNATIVE TREATMENTS

Besides managing the complications of sickle cell disease as they occur, the only other current alternatives to hydroxyurea therapy are:

1. regular transfusions
2. bone marrow transplantation (You will find a detailed review of bone marrow transplant in "New treatments and Research", Chapter 15 in Part III.)

Both of these alternatives have major risks as well as major benefits. Talk with your doctor about how these balance for your child.

Still other treatments for sickle cell disease are in the research pipeline, but none is likely to be available outside of a clinical research trial for a couple of years.

GUIDE FOR TEACHERS

It is a good idea to meet with your child's teachers and find out what they know about sickle cell disease. If there is a school nurse let her or him know about your child. Most sickle cell clinics have a handout to give teachers. You can help educate your teachers. Here is a sample guide you can modify to your special needs.

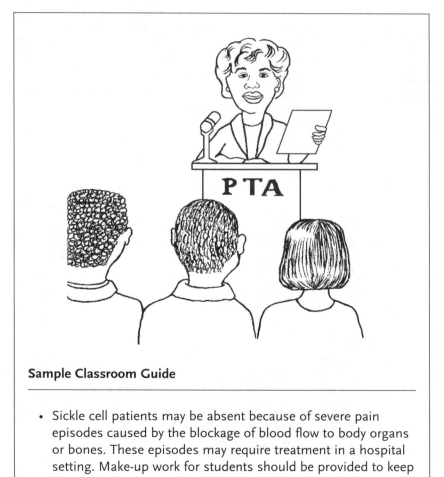

Sample Classroom Guide

- Sickle cell patients may be absent because of severe pain episodes caused by the blockage of blood flow to body organs or bones. These episodes may require treatment in a hospital setting. Make-up work for students should be provided to keep the student current with assignments. A hospital- or home-based teacher may be required for prolonged complications.

- Pain episodes may be prevented by allowing persons with sickle cell disease to keep well hydrated with water. Let them keep a water bottle with them or allow frequent water breaks. They will require frequent bathroom breaks also because their kidneys cannot retain water as well as normal kidneys do.
- Pain episodes may also be prevented by not allowing the individual to become over-heated or exposed to cold temperatures.
- Because of their anemia, individuals with sickle cell may tire before others and a rest period may be appropriate.
- Encourage gym and sports participation but because of anemia, persons with sickle cell may tire before others. Allow them to stop and take breaks without undue attention.
- Sickle cell disease does not affect one's intelligence, but various effects of this lifelong illness may impair academic performance. These should be identified and addressed, as they would for any child. Academic performance is especially important now that life expectancy for those with sickle cell is up in the fourth and fifth decade. Those with sickle cell, as well as anyone, can become professionals like doctors, engineers, and lawyers.
- Sickle cell patients may have a yellow tint to their eyes because of the anemia, this is not usually a liver problem. They also may have a shorter stature and delayed puberty.
- Students with sickle cell should be treated as normally as possible, with an awareness that they may have intermittent episodes of pain, infection or fatigue that can be treated and sometimes prevented through adequate water intake, avoiding temperature extremes and overdoing it.
- Learn about sickle cell and understand the challenges that students with this disease must face.
- Have a plan of action with the individual to do what you can to keep them productive and complication free.

Medical attention is needed when any of the following occur:
- fever
- headache
- chest pain
- abdominal pain
- numbness or weakness.

A mild pain episode may be managed with increased fluid intake and a non-narcotic pain pill like ibuprofen or acetaminophen.

Your school can launch a sickle cell awareness program by encouraging activities like these:

- Invite a speaker from your local sickle cell foundation or clinic to educate the entire class or staff about sickle cell.
- Become involved in public awareness events like walks, fun runs, kids' camp and fund raisers.
- Encourage blood donations and blood drives in your community. Many with sickle cell need transfusions to prevent childhood strokes and other complications.
- Support sickle cell research to provide new treatments.
- Encourage sickle cell patients to be the best they can be.

CHAPTER 10

Teenage: 13 to 18 Years

HEIDY'S STORY

For as long as I can remember I have longed to be normal, and sometimes that longing made my life even harder than it was already. I was ashamed to be ill, and sometimes angry that pain episodes and other medical problems kept me from living what to me seemed the free and easy lives of my friends.

But when I was ten, in the hospital for treatment for one of my many pain episodes, something clicked. I sat up in bed and told myself I'd never feel sorry for myself again.

The way I remember coming to that insight and resolution was this. I'd been hospitalized over 100 times for pain episodes. I understood what caused the pain, but that didn't make the trips to the emergency room any easier. I knew the treatment. Strong drugs like morphine and Demerol and fluid given to me intravenously.

I hated the trips to the emergency room, even though without them I couldn't get rid of the pain. Sometimes the pain was OK, sometimes I felt as if I were about to die. Month after month, I'd have one of these crises, and I'd pray to God for an answer to the question I never stopped asking, "Why me?"

Sometimes when I was a child I'd ignore the limits the doctors had warned me about. I'd swim in the school pool, even though I'd sometimes get sick afterwards because the water was too cold. I was trying very hard to kid myself. I actually believed for a while that if I didn't think of myself as being sick I wouldn't be, so I ignored many warnings and tried hard to hide my sickness from friends and family

That went on for years, and during that time I wasn't doing very well as a patient. But by now I was older and a little more open to reason. My doctors told me that I would be able to deal with sickle cell disease only if I learned about it. So I did learn.

As I got older I understood that sometimes I had to deal with doctors and nurses who didn't know much about sickle cell disease. I made it my business to educate them, by telling them patiently about the illness and about what I needed to make my symptoms more manageable. I began to follow the research, and to know about the people and clinics searching for a cure. To sum it all up, as a child I was afraid to tell the truth about who I really was. I was afraid even to know that truth. Now I accept it and let other people know because I realize that, for the while at least, sickle cell disease is part of me.

Today I can honestly say that in a way sickle cell has become a blessing. It has made me stronger by making me come to terms with myself. I know I'm one of the lucky ones. There are some people out there with this disease who lack the help they need. I have a loving and understanding family. Even though they can not feel my pain, they are with me every step of the way. As for friends, they come and go but there are some I have had since childhood who cry every time they see me in pain. I am thankful for them.

My quest for normalcy has faded into a devotion to aid, as much as I can, those with my disease. I am now at the beginning of a new quest to find a cure for my disease.

COMMON MANIFESTATIONS

As Heidy could tell you, each stage of maturation brings new problems and the need for new solutions. Adolescence can be hard on anyone, but it is especially hard on people with sickle cell disease. A broad range of physical ailments can, and does occur.

AUTO-SPLENECTOMY

The previously enlarged spleen begins to shrink as a result of tissue death caused by inadequate blood supply. As a result of this shrinkage (called *infarction*), the spleen may disappear entirely by the end of adolescence. (Doctors call this *auto-splenectomy*— literally, the body performing a *splenectomy*, or spleen removal on itself.) While the teenager can live without a spleen, it does have important immune functions; without it the patient will probably experience more infections. These infections, in turn, increase the risk of more crises.

PRIAPISM

In males with sickle cell diseases, priapism, or painful prolonged erections of the penis, may occur as a result of sickled cells blocking the outflow of blood from the penis. This problem is more frequent in uncircumcised boys because the foreskin acts like an elastic band around the penis. Circumcision will often partially correct the problem. Repeated episodes of priapism can, unfortunately, lead to permanent impotence.

CHRONIC ULCERS

Chronic ulcers may form, especially on or near the inner side of the ankles. They result from blockage of the blood supply to the skin by sickled red blood cells and other material. The ulcers generally appear pale with a yellowish tinge. They are difficult to heal, even with the help of surgical interventions .

CHRONIC BONE INFECTIONS

Chronic bone infections with chronically discharging openings are all too common. These bone infections (known as osteomyelitis) are difficult to cure. Sometimes they require months of intravenous and/or oral antibiotic therapy, often combined with localized surgery.

DELAYED PUBERTY

Puberty in children with sickle cell disease is sometimes delayed, as it is in children with other debilitating, chronic illnesses. For girls, the onset of the first menstrual period (or *menarche)* and breast development may both be late. In boys, the testicles remain small longer and body hair growth may be delayed.

EMOTIONAL PROBLEMS

Emotional problems result from trying to deal with the over-whelming range of problems—the fatigue, bouts of acute illness, pain, fear of death, and social isolation. Depression is common and can be treated by professional counselors. School grades can fall. Drug abuse may occur as a way of coping with physical and emotional pain.

PREVENTIVE MEASURES

Patients and parents will already be familiar with the best ways to prevent pain—a set of guidelines known as FARMS. See p. 112–113 for a discussion of these guidelines.

NO SMOKING, NO ALCOHOL, NO DRUGS

Smoking robs the red cells of oxygen. Alcohol dehydrates the body and can damage the liver over time. Alcohol can also make the blood more acidic and this can cause sickling. Finally, alcohol impairs judgment and can lead to mistakes.

Illegal drugs like cocaine can kill people without sickle cell and are much more dangerous in those with it.

BIRTH CONTROL OPTIONS—SEXUALITY

Parents should counsel teens about the benefits of abstinence and monogamous relationships. But if the teen is sexually active, prevention against HIV and sexually transmitted diseases is critical.

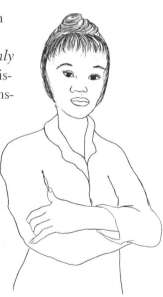

- The combination of a latex condom and spermicidal foam provides safe, effective contraception and *is the only method* that may reduce the transmission of AIDS and other sexually transmitted diseases.
- Oral contraception is probably the most effective method and is probably safe if low-dose estrogen preparations are used.
- The IUD is also effective, though with this form of contraception there is increased risk of infection.
- Diaphragms are usually less effective, but may be satisfactory if combined with a spermicidal preparation.
- Progesterone based prevention by pill or depo injection preparations is also effective.

It is critically important to know that oral contraception, IUDs, diaphragms, or progesterone will NOT protect you against HIV/AIDs.

CLINICAL ISSUES

- Discuss sexual development and issues with your child.
- Assist your child in progressing to independence, stressing self-management coping skills, and academic achievement.
- Discuss with your child birth control, prevention of complications, learning physical limits, sexually transmitted disease, and substance abuse.
- Provide peer support by encouraging support group contact and activities.
- Discuss realistic job and career goals and college.
- Schedule clinic visits every four to six months.

PSYCHO-SOCIAL ISSUES
TEEN ISSUES

Teens should be counseled about all of the dangers facing other teens. Teens with sickle cell are at higher risk of injury or death from guns, auto accidents, suicide, drugs and alcohol, than from their disease. Encourage seat belt use, avoiding alcohol, avoiding those with guns and street drugs. Risky sexual behavior can lead to HIV and other sexually transmitted diseases. It is important to spend time with teens affirming and supporting them. Supportive friends and parents can be positive influences.

Explore the symptoms of depression or drug abuse, including sleep disturbances, eating disorders, lack of interest in favorite activities, and withdrawal from friends and family. Ask about suicidal thoughts and plans. These should be taken very seriously and professional help sought immediately if such plans are revealed.

PUBERTY

Puberty may be delayed by two to three years in those with sickle cell disease. Teens and parents should be assured that puberty will occur. With the onset of puberty come emotional highs and lows.

Self-esteem may suffer when one's peers are growing and developing secondary sex characteristics, and you are doing so at a much slower rate.

TRANSITION TO ADULT HEALTH CARE TEAM

It is important to make the transition from pediatric services to adult caregivers over a period of time. The treatment philosophy is quite different in a children's hospital from that of an adult inpatient ward. Take time to get to know the adult doctors, nurses, and social workers. Learn about all of the adult services available. Some centers offer teen clinics to meet the special needs of adolescents.

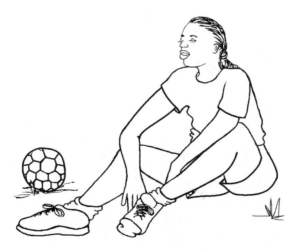

CHAPTER 11

Young Adult: 19 to 25 years

MELISSA'S STORY

My name is Melissa Creary and I want to dispel the myths about sickle cell disease and the West Indian culture. I was three years old when I was diagnosed with sickle cell disease. It was a beautiful summer day, and I was playing in the backyard wading pool, while my mother and father chatted nearby. That night I was restless and ill, and nothing seemed to calm me.

In the morning my parents took me to our family doctor, and he arranged for me to have some tests, which led to more tests. At one point, the doctors thought I had leukemia. It was not until my aunt, a nurse, asked my mother if I had ever been tested for sickle cell anemia, that my family finally glimpsed the answer. The test showed that this was just what I had.

Both of my parents had emigrated from Jamaica to the United States and although the disease is common in Jamaica, unfortunately neither of them had even heard of it. They didn't know that they each carried a gene for altered hemoglobin, which left them untouched but had a drastic effect on my own genetic make-up. The hemoglobin portion of my red blood cells (the part that carries oxygen to all of my body parts) was changed so that sometimes it caused my normal blood cells to sickle. My parents were told that I had the SC variant.

I learned lessons the hard way. For example, the kids in our fifth grade gym class were expected to run a mile. Instead of telling my instructor that I was tired, I pushed myself to exhaustion. I completed the run but I missed the rest of the school year.

The strains that triggered episodes weren't always physical. During my junior year in college, I was so stressed out about a test that I ended up in the ER.

I was hospitalized only twice during my adolescence. The fact is that the disease, in whatever form, does not affect everybody in the same way or with the same severity.

Learning about the sickle cell trait was very important to me, since that trait had so much to do with who I am. In Jamaica about 10% of the population has the sickle cell trait, but in other islands the frequency varies from 7% in Barbados to as high as 13% to 14% in Dominica and St. Lucia. This compares to about 8% in the Black American population, and frequencies of 20% to 30% in Black populations of West Africa and of some populations in Saudi Arabia, India, Greece, and Italy.

So it's important to find out if you carry the sickle cell gene by getting a simple and painless blood test called hemoglobin electrophoresis. I think everybody who comes from one of those population groups ought to have that test, but especially pregnant women or people thinking of having a child. Getting tested is easy. Tests can be arranged by your general practitioner or at your local sickle cell center or foundation. Soon, nearly everyone will be screened at birth. Newborn screening is mandatory. Even today most states will require newborn screening.

When I was three, there wasn't much going on in sickle cell research or treatments. Twenty years later, the outlook for someone like me who has the disease has improved tremendously. In the past, survival beyond the age of thirty was unlikely. Now it's common for many of us with the disease to live well beyond that age.

There's still plenty of work to be done. In my community, and many others, access to medical care can be difficult for a lot of people, but improvements are occurring as people learn more and more about how to find the medical help they need.

You may have guessed already, but I am now involved in researching sickle cell disease to try to improve the quality of life of those whom it affects. I've made this my life's work.

Where there's ignorance, there's myth, and myths surround sickle cell disease. So let's dispel some of those myths about a disease that annually affects 50,000 Blacks in the United States alone.

- Sickle cell disease is not contagious; it is a genetic disorder you receive from birth.
- It is not cancer.
- The mind is not affected. (I completed a college degree, am working, and will be going to graduate school next year.)
- It is not just a "Black" disease but affects Hispanics and people of Asian and Mediterranean origin as well.
- It is not "bad blood" or a family curse.

Sickle cell is a disease that exists just as any other except in a way unlike any other. In its uniqueness, it offers challenges to both those who treat it and those who live with it. It is a disease that has molded my life and made me who I am and hope to be.

COMMON MANIFESTATIONS
LEG ULCERS

Leg ulcers cause chronic disability in 10% to 15% of older children and young adults with sickle cell anemia. Leg ulcers in those with sickle cell diseases start as a result of localized tissue death in the skin, which in turn is caused by clogging of small blood vessels with sickled red blood cells and blood clot.

Treatment includes:

- Medication. It has been reported that Trental™ is helpful in healing some kinds of leg ulcers and it is possible that it may also speed the healing of sickle cell leg ulcers. A newer drug,

Pletal™ (cilostazol) may also be helpful. Healing of many skin ulcers may be accelerated by applying a compound called becaplermin (Regranex). This gel is applied sparingly, directly to the ulcer, and covered with a clean gauze pad moistened with saline solution—available from the pharmacy without prescription as "irrigation saline."

- Good nutrition.
- Removing dead tissue. This speeds healing and prevents infection. It is done using dressings like Duoderm™.
- Grafting. When leg ulcers cannot be healed by any other means, surgical skin grafting may need to be performed.
- A bioengineered temporary skin substitute called Apligraft™.
- Taking oral zinc sulfate.
- Using wet/dry dressings
- Bed rest and leg elevation
- Using a zinc impregnated bandage or unna boot two-three times per week.
- Blood transfusion therapy.

AVASCULAR NECROSIS OF THE HIPS AND SHOULDERS

The round part of the hip bone and shoulder bone each have one artery supplying blood flow to keep the bone alive and healthy. This artery can be blocked by sickle red blood cells. If this happens it could cause the round end of the bone to die. This condition, avascular necrosis, is most common in Hb SC and S beta tha-lassemia type sickle cell disease.

In a patient with avascular necrosis the affected area begins to collapse, making the round ball shape turn rough and jagged. This causes pain when walking or moving the leg at the hip joint and in the arm in the shoulder joint.

The first line of treatment is to use daily arthritis medications that are safe (see the chronic pain treatment section). But the long range objective is to prevent further joint destruction by taking weight off the hip by using a cane, or crutch, and by limiting walking. The shoulder is rested as much as possible. A physical therapist can help teach you how to exercise without damaging the joint further.

Once the pain level becomes too high and can't be controlled with medications or physical limits, a visit to the orthopedic surgeon for a consultation about a joint replacement should be scheduled. There are artificial hips and shoulders, but they last only about ten years with moderate use. Because sickle cell patients are living longer, one can expect a hip replaced at age twenty to be replaced again at ages thirty, forty and fifty.

The risk of joint replacement is post-operative complications, joint infection, and joint failure. The surgeon should work with your doctor to insure the safest possible surgery with a preoperative blood transfusion to raise your hemoglobin to 10, indicating good hydration, and incentive spirometry (blow bottles) after surgery.

PREGNANCY

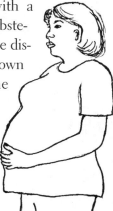

Management of pregnancy in the patient with a sickle syndrome requires coordinated care by obstetricians and hematologists knowledgeable in the disease. Although complications have gone down over the last twenty years, there are still some increased risks for both mother and child. With careful management, there is no reason that women with sickle syndromes cannot have children.

All sickle cell patients should receive accurate information at puberty and periodically throughout their reproductive lives about the risks of pregnancy, genetic transmission of sickle syndromes, methods of contraception, prenatal diagnosis, prevention of sexually transmitted disease and the increased responsibility of raising children.

All pregnant patients should be under the care of an obstetrician with interest and expertise in managing pregnancy in sickle syndrome patients. The primary care physician and hematologist should also be involved as members of the management team.

Most pregnant patients should be on folic acid, prenatal vitamins, and standard iron supplementation unless iron overload is present. Follow-up visits are usually scheduled every two weeks, with weekly visits when necessary for complications, and during the last four to six weeks of the pregnancy.

EYE PROBLEMS

Blocked blood flow in the small blood vessels in the back of the eye causes the eye to make new, weaker, blood vessels to bypass the blocked ones. These new blood vessels are thinner and tend to break open, causing bleeding into the clear eye fluid. This can also cause the retina, the seeing part of the eye, to detach. The result can be blindness.

Patients with Hb SC disease, and perhaps sickle thalassemias, are at increased risk for these eye complications. Yearly eye examination by an eye doctor, with appropriate use of laser surgery, if necessary, may reduce the severity of these complications.

PREVENTIVE MEASURES

In this age group, the FARMS include:

F—Fluids. Drink 8–10 glasses of water a day and daily folate, 1mg.

Air—Avoiding altitudes, smoking and asthma

Rest when you need to and don't overdo physical activity

M—Medications like hydrea may be the best preventive

Situations to avoid: temperature extremes, alcohol, illegal drugs

CLINICAL ISSUES

- Schedule clinic visits for a history, physical, CBC, every 2 to 6 months. A reticulocyte count, and urinalysis should be done at each visit. Get blood chemistries, an eye exam, and a PPD skin test once a year. Screen for gallstones and aseptic necrosis if symptoms occur.
- Learn all about your sickle disease, pain management, prevention of complications, response to emergencies, and avoiding substance abuse.
- Learn the importance of knowing your limits, hydration, diet, and dental care.
- Ask your provider about disease variability, prognosis, and prospects for future therapy.
- Seek psycho-social support when needed.
- Learn how to do breast or testicle self examination.

PSYCHO-SOCIAL ISSUES

Young adulthood brings new challenges to everyone and, as always, the challenges will be especially strong for people with sickle cell disease. Three of the new challenges are career choice, raising one's own family, and knowing how to accept and even seek the support of others.

CAREER CHOICES

You'll want to avoid jobs that could make your sickle cell disease worse. These tend to be outdoor jobs with exposure to temperature fluctuations, or manual labor that can cause fatigue and increased sickling. Standing for long periods may cause pain in the hips and knees in areas with blocked blood flow and bone damage.

We recommend jobs that are indoors, that are not manual, that have good health insurance benefits, and that are enjoyable. We encourage patients to work hard in school and try to go to college or vocational school.

It is good to work for an employer that understands sickle cell disease and knows that you may sometimes have to miss work because of pain events or other complications. A letter from your doctor with information we have outlined in this book is a good first start.

FAMILY ISSUES

Many family members with sickle cell disease choose to live near parents, or brothers and sisters, who can help them when they need transportation, child sitting, help with household chores, and support when complications or severe pain episodes occur. Often, for the family, this is a continuation of a support system long developed.

PEER SUPPORT

A successful patient's network will reach beyond the family to other patients, with whom one can offer and receive support and ideas, encourage and be encouraged, help raise community awareness, and advocate for excellent care in the local health care facilities. Monthly meetings at a local home, meeting room at the library or hospital can help keep all informed about the latest news in the community. Communicate with newsletters, phone chains, email, and even websites.

CHAPTER 12

Adulthood: 26 to 40 years

MICHELLE'S STORY

My name is Michelle Rodriguez. I was born in Brooklyn, N. Y., and I am thirty-one years old. I was born with sickle cell disease. My parents both had the sickle cell trait, though they didn't suffer from the disease. But they did have trouble with diabetes, heart disease, and high blood pressure that ran in both their families.

I don't remember much about how sickle cell struck me in early childhood, but when I was ten my mother told me that I had stayed in the hospital for two months after I was born while the doctors gave me blood transfusions and other kinds of IV treatment.

As a young child I often had sickle cell attacks, and these attacks got worse as I got older. I did what I could with folic acid.

I didn't do very well. My pain was often terrible and I grew weaker. My schooling was interrupted and almost ended by the disease. In junior high school, for instance, I missed two to three months of school each year.

I tried hard to keep my life normal. I got through junior high by going to summer school for an extra semester. I was lucky to have a loving mother who taught me never to give up.

By the time I got to high school the attacks got less frequent and less severe. I got through my freshman year very well. Then, in the beginning of my sophomore year, I got pregnant. As bad as this can be for any young girl, it was especially bad for me. During my pregnancy I was in and out of the hospital all the time. I suffered severe joint pains and from an infection the doctors couldn't pinpoint.

When it came time for the delivery of the child, I was in crisis. I was suffering such severe joint pains and labor pains at the same time that I was never moved to the delivery room. Hooked to an IV and monitoring machines, torn by the double sets of pain that ran through me, I continued this terrible labor until, finally, the doctors had to deliver the baby by Caesarian section.

I first saw my baby in the nursery, and wanted to cry. She weighed only two pounds and five ounces, and it broke my heart to see this little infant already hooked to so many machines. I didn't think she'd live.

I'm happy to say that Dominique *did* live. Maybe she inherited that same courage my mother had taught me. I went on to graduate from high school. My sickle cell attacks became much rarer and less severe after my pregnancy. But shortly after I graduated, I had to have surgery, and when I was recovering the sickle cell attacks grew worse, and I was in and out of the hospital again.

That's when I met a doctor who told me about a new medicine, Trental™, that might help me. He didn't make any promises and told me not to get my hopes too high, but he thought it was worth a try. I agreed. I didn't want to have my life stopped over and over again by hospital stays.

So I started to take the new medication and it took my body more than a year to respond. But gradually I noticed changes: I was less tired, I rarely had joint pains and when I did they were less severe. I managed to stay out of the hospital, except for one occasion, and even that was far less serious than the previous attacks that brought me to the hospital.

I think mine is a happy story. Much of my suffering is behind me, and finally I can say proudly that I have learned to live with sickle cell disease.

COMMON MANIFESTATIONS

BONE PAIN

At this age, more prolonged and constant pain can be seen with bone infarction, sickle arthritis, and aseptic necrosis of the hip bone or shoulder. With chronic pain, the safest non-steroidal anti-inflammatory medications should be given. Trans-cutaneous electrical nerve stimulation (TENS) units, relaxation techniques, occupational and physical therapy approaches may be useful in reducing pain and maintaining a functional lifestyle. Education and support are often required to prevent addiction to the drugs that may be used to control the pain.

KIDNEY PROBLEMS

Kidney damage starts very early and progresses throughout life. With advancing age, protein in the urine and kidney damage may occur. All patients should be screened for protein in the urine annually beginning at age thirteen. If the kidneys stops working, poisons are not filtered out of the blood and you can become very ill.

The next step is dialysis—running your blood through a kidney machine or peritoneal dialysis. Peritoneal dialysis involves putting a filtering solution in the abdomen, letting it stay for awhile to remove the body's poisons, then draining the solution. This form of dialysis can be done at home three to four times a week by the individual or family members.

LUNG PROBLEMS

Pneumonias, acute chest syndrome caused by red cell sickling in lung blood vessels, and fat from bone marrow blockage, are acute complications seen with increased frequency in patients with sickle syndromes. They are sometimes hard to diagnose because signs of chest pain, cough, fever, pulmonary infiltrates, and severe hypoxia are common to all. Reactive airway disease is common and may be more prevalent in patients with sickle cell disease.

Treatment for lung problems includes hospitalization with careful monitoring of hemoglobin and blood gasses, oxygen for hypoxia, IV hydration and pain treatment, antibiotics, and exchange transfusion in episodes with severe hypoxia, rapid progression, or diffuse pulmonary involvement.

Chest syndrome may be prevented by the use of incentive spirometry in all hospitalized patients. Older patients may develop chronic restrictive lung disease, pulmonary hypertension, and cor pulmonale. If the oxygen level is always low, then home oxygen may be prescribed to aid breathing.

PREVENTIVE MEASURES

In addition to normal FARMS prevention, men and women of this age should participate in cancer screening, including mammograms and PAP smears for women, and prostate screening in males.

PSYCHO-SOCIAL ISSUES

Missing work, family pressures, depression, insomnia and anxiety are the most common social issues in this age group. A professional counselor, social worker, clergy member, or psychiatrist can be a great benefit in managing them. There are medications that help depression and help treat chronic pain at the same time. A psychiatrist or your primary care doctor can prescribe these medications.

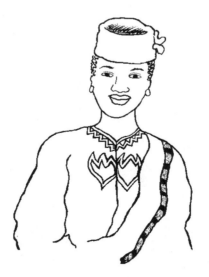

PEER SUPPORT

Meeting with other adults with sickle cell disease can help you relieve stress, share resources, and provide coping ideas for the pressures of life. The fellowship of other sickle cell patients can help build self-esteem and improve hope. Invite special speakers to address issues common to all. Get involved; volunteer to be a role model for younger patients.

CHAPTER 13

Adults Over Forty

INGRID'S STORY

My name is Ingrid Whittaker-Ware, Esq. I was born in 1962 to Raphael and Muriel Whittaker, and was the fourth of five children. I was raised on the sunny island of Jamaica and emigrated to Atlanta, Georgia in 1980.

I was diagnosed with sickle cell disease (SS) at eleven months old. Although I had signs of jaundice from birth, the doctors did not properly diagnose my disease until I was having an uncontrolled fever and crying more than usual for an eleven month old. I am the only one of my siblings to be born with the disease. Both my parents have the sickle trait, as do one brother and my little sister.

My parents taught me as a child the value and empowerment of knowledge and determination. Once when I was having a pain episode, I cried and begged my parents to send me to school. I wanted this so badly that they let me go. That same day, during the lunch hour, I was hit in the head by a stray stone thrown by someone on the playground. The teachers wanted to call my parents right away, but I begged them not to, because I feared my parents would take me home and keep me out of school for several days until I was completely well.

At that time, being in school helped to lift my spirits and take my mind off being more physically challenged than my peers.

I was blessed to have had the expert and compassionate care of Drs. Elaine Reid and Graham Serjeant. To them both I owe a depth of gratitude for the care they provided me while I was growing up. But then, I have been blessed from the time I was born. When I was diagnosed with sickle cell disease, the doctors did not expect me to live past my sixth birthday. In fact, at first I was diagnosed as having leukemia, and it was not until further testing that the doctors came up with the diagnosis of sickle cell disease.

Despite the gloomy predictions from the doctors, the good Lord is the author of my life and had other plans for me. So, He has always placed me in the care of the very best doctors in the area of sickle cell disease and research. Dr. Reid watched over me the only two times I was hospitalized as a child. The first of those two times I was not expected to live because of the seriousness of the infection. I was very young then and do not remember much about that hospitalization, but I do remember being placed in an oxygen tent and the grim expressions of the medical staff and my parents. I survived then as I am surviving now. Dr. Serjeant cared for me through adolescence into adulthood, and it was he who first taught me to protect my legs from insect bites and injuries in an effort to minimize leg ulcers.

I attended Spelman College and graduated with a double major in three and a half years. At Spelman I majored in political science and economics with a minor in international relations. I graduated *magna cum laude*. Life at Spelman was fun. My professors inspired and challenged me to reach for the stars and further instilled in me the conviction that knowledge is power. For the most part, I stayed out of trouble with sickle cell disease at Spelman, although there were stressful times, what with the pressure of exams and the like. I viewed that type of stress as a positive challenge and managed never to have a serious pain episode for which I had to be hospitalized. I tried my best to take care of myself by hydrating myself constantly and follow the healthy practices I learned early in life, and which were reinforced by the staff at the Grady Sickle Cell Center.

I had several leg ulcers, and one bout with what was suspected to be osteomyelitis while I was at Spelman. I remember my mother waking me up early one morning and asking why I was moaning. I told her that I was not moaning, but then immediately felt the pain in my ankle. This was the first time I was given a mild narcotic medication (Tylenol 3) to help control the pain. I could not do my usual activities that summer, which included working at a summer job. However, I refused to let the summer be an entire loss and decided to take a course in calligraphy. I am still able to write calligraphy today and sometimes get requests from family members to do a special piece for them. At Spelman I also took time for piano lessons again, which I hadn't done since I was a child. Playing music, particularly the piano, often helped me relax and reduced my stress.

At Spelman I won the prestigious Thomas Watson Fellowship. This fellowship gave me the chance to travel to Venezuela, in Latin America, and extensively in Europe, in the quest of being a "better world citizen." On returning from my travels, in 1985, I enrolled in Columbia University School of Law in New York City. I graduated from Columbia and returned to Atlanta to work as an attorney for the federal government, where I have been for the last thirteen years.

Whether I travel on business or for pleasure, I always take care to properly hydrate myself before, during, and after flying and have never encountered any major sickle cell related problems due to air pressure. The air does sometimes become a little dry, but I counter that by breathing into a cup with a few drops of water or a few slices of lemon. A flight attendant taught me that trick while I was on one of the long flights from the United States to Venezuela, when the dry air had become uncomfortable to breathe.

During my life's journey, I have had many challenges, particularly in the last seven or eight years, as I have grown older. However, I have also had God's protection and His many blessings. Some of my challenges from sickle cell disease have included recurrent and painful leg ulcers and one aplastic crisis. The aplastic crisis racked my body with so much pain that I can only describe it as feeling like I had been hit by a runaway freight train. This aplastic episode was also accompanied by high fevers in excess of 105 degrees. I remember awaking from a feverish sleep to see my husband shivering with cold as he sat in the room with me. The doctors had severely lowered the room temperature to try to bring my body temperature down. I also have frequent pain episodes (which thankfully I usually do not have to be hospitalized for), mild retinopathy, and frequent blood transfusions (a fairly recent development). In addition I had gall bladder disease and a heart attack before age forty. I have also had other illnesses which were not initially sickle cell related, but became so when sickle related complications developed.

Despite the bleak outlook and shortened life expectancy predicted by doctors when I was first diagnosed with the disease, I am here to tell my story almost four decades later. I have also been blessed with a very supportive family, including a mother and father who had faith that their first daughter would survive and did everything in their power to ensure that I did. Their efforts included making sure they learned as much as they could about the disease and then passing that knowledge on to me so that I could, in turn, take care of myself. My parents maintained appropriate communications with my doctors while I was a child so that I could get proper and immediate treatment when necessary; ensured I had a proper diet and nutrition; and provided a comfortable, positive and stable environment in which I could grow up. My three brothers, sister and extended family and friends have also always been very supportive of me.

Today, I am married to Willie J. Ware, Jr., my caring and supportive husband, who stands guard at my bedside each time I am ill. He hovers over me like a mother hen and gets on my case about taking care of myself as much as, or worse than, my mother does. I am also the proud mother of the cutest and most charming three year old toddler, William, who came into our family by adoption. I am fulfilled by having the joy and comfort of knowing that I am loved and cared about by not only my husband and son, but by my extended family and friends as well.

To my comrades in arms who live with the disease, I challenge you to:

- Develop your spiritual life and ask for God's continued blessings, because even when the doctors and everyone else give up hope, He is the only one that can bring you through the many trials that you face.
- Adopt a positive attitude and know that with God's help you can do anything you put your mind to—believe in yourself.
- Believe that knowledge is indeed power and educate yourself as much as you can about your disease and your body and take all the steps necessary to stay healthy and positive, including maintaining proper contacts with your health care providers and maintaining a healthy diet.
- Continue to have faith and hope that a cure to this disease will be found soon, and do whatever you can to contribute to that cause.

To caregivers, family and friends I say thank you and continue to keep the faith. Keep yourself and your loved ones encouraged. The more you learn about the disease the more you can help your loved ones and educate others in the fight against sickle cell disease. To health care professionals, again I say thank you. I also challenge you to continue to provide care in a compassionate fashion, treating your patients with the respect and dignity you would accord anyone who comes across your path. You never know—you could be entertaining a future lawyer, doctor or influential person. Encourage your patients to live as full and productive a life as possible.

COMMON MANIFESTATIONS
MENOPAUSE

There are no reported research articles about menopause in sickle cell patients. At the same time, we have seen clinically that women have more pain events and complications during this time period. Estrogen replacement may or may not be beneficial. Check with your doctor to determine what's right for you.

PREVENTIVE MEASURES

In this age group, the FARMS or preventive measures are the same as in chapter 12.

PSYCHO-SOCIAL ISSUES AND SUPPORT

While adults will continue to benefit from peer support and support on the job, they will also be able, on the strength of their experiences, to help others in their practical and spiritual struggles. There is much you can do for yourself and for others:

- Develop hobbies and interests to distract yourself from daily pain.
- Get involved with fund raising, or volunteering in the hospital.
- Become a mentor to a child or teen with sickle cell disease. Help others with school work.
- Be a camp counselor.
- Be a public speaker in your community.
- Get involved with politics to improve services for sickle cell patients.

This is a time to share your wisdom with the younger generation.

SPIRITUAL ISSUES

Patients with a solid spiritual foundation seem to do better physically and emotionally and are less depressive. Become involved in your local place of worship. People with a solid spiritual foundation experience less stress and fear of death. They also have a community of support when they are ill to help with family issues, transportation, meals, counseling, and encouragement.

PART THREE

LIVING WITH
SICKLE CELL DISEASE

CHAPTER 14

Pain Assessment and Pain Management

INTRODUCTION

Of the many symptoms that can torment sickle cell patients, pain is one of the most common and distressing. This chapter tells you what you need to know about

- The causes of pain
- Pain prevention
- Home treatment
- Emergency treatment
- Inpatient treatment in the hospital.

We can't repeat it too often: *knowledge is power*. The more one knows about the causes, prevention and treatment of pain, the better the chances of an early recovery. Certain types and causes of pain require a clinician's help and advice about treatment. Until recently, a doctor's assessment of a patient's pain could be quite subjective, and patients who were suffering were sometimes made to feel as if they were malingering, or even exaggerating pain in order to get drugs. Today, the Joint Commission on Accreditation of Healthcare Organizations (JCAHO), the agency that inspects and certifies all US hospitals, has issued new standards for pain assessment, treatment and education. These new pain management standards should improve the pain care sickle cell patients receive.

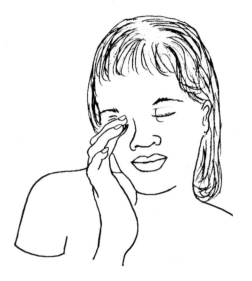

The most common acute problem of sickle cell disease is the sickle pain episode (also unfortunately termed pain "crisis"). A pain episode is defined as "a self-limited episode of diffuse, reversible pain often occurring in the extremities, back, chest, and abdomen." The severity of pain can range from mild attacks of five minutes to excruciating pain lasting days or weeks and requiring hospitalization. This intense pain is believed to be caused by the inflammatory response to bone or marrow death, or necrosis, reduced blood flow, or ischemia, ischemic muscle, and ischemic bowel resulting from the obstruction and sludging of blood flow produced by sickled red blood cells, or erythrocytes.

Although the pain episode is almost never a cause of death, affected individuals often fear serious complications or death. The frequency of pain episode varies with each person, depending upon his or her hemoglobin phenotype, physical condition, and many other variables. Trigger factors include events that cause increased physical and psychological stress, especially fever, dehydration, overexertion, rapid temperature change, or anger. Episodes, however, frequently occur without any apparent causes.

The management of a pain episode begins with a complete clinical evaluation to exclude life-threatening complications, and to identify causes of pain that are not related to sickle cell disease. A detailed history and physical examination allows the doctor to identify treatable factors such as infection, dehydration, acidosis from any cause, emotional stress, extreme temperature exposure, or ingestion of other substances such as alcohol or other recreational drugs.

Since there are no characteristic findings that define the severity of a pain episode, *the patient's assessment must be accepted.* Treatment of a pain episode includes oral or intravenous hydration, analgesics, bed rest, and treatment of the underlying causes, such as infection.

RECORDING PAIN

It helps you and your health care providers to record the following information about your pain in a daily diary. Use the acronym **LOCATES** to locate the pain:

L—Location. Note the exact location of the pain and describe if it "travels" anywhere.

O—Other Symptoms. Record any other symptoms like fever, nausea, cough, that comes with the pain.

C—Character. Describe the pain. Is it deep? burning? throbbing? Other?

A—Aggravating and Alleviating Things. What makes the pain better and what makes the pain worse?

T—Timing. When did the pain start, has it been there all the time, or does it come and go?

E—Environment and Effect. Where were you and what were you doing when the pain started. How does the pain affect your daily routine?

S—Severity. Be honest. If you always overstate your pain score, thinking health care providers will not treat you with enough pain medication, it could lead you to be over medicated and have more side effects. Develop a sense of trust with your health care providers. They need to believe you and treat your stated level of pain with the appropriate amount of medication.

Pain scales should be available in the ER and the hospital. A scale you should be familiar with is the Visual Analog Scale or VAS. It is a 10 centimeter line with numbers from 0 to 10. 0 is "no pain" and 10 is "the worst pain you have ever had in your life." Mark on the line where you would rate your level of pain.

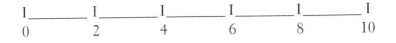

I_____ I_____ I_____ I_____ I_____ I
0   2   4   6   8   10

PAIN PREVENTION

For general pain prevention remember FARMS.

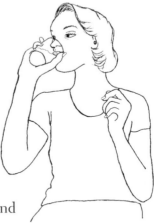

TYPES OF PAIN

There are five identifiable types of pain, each with different treatments.

1. Acute sickle cell pain episode—pain that can last for several minutes to several days, caused by blocked blood flow from the sickle red blood cells. This pain is usually deep in the bones and muscles of the arms, legs, and back. Pain in the head, chest, or belly or pain with fever should be immediately evaluated by a health care provider.

2. Acute pain from another cause—pain that comes on suddenly and feels different from your usual pain episode should be checked by your health care provider. Pain in sickle cell

patients may have other causes, such as stomach
ulcers, appendicitis, a slipped disk, menstrual
cramps, and so forth.

3. Chronic pain from sickle cell bone damage—pain that lasts longer than a few
weeks and may be present daily. This
occurs when bones are damaged by
the blocked blood flow.

4. Chronic pain from other causes—daily
pain that lasts more than six weeks
caused by such things as a slipped disk,
rheumatoid arthritis, old injuries, and so
forth.

5. Chronic nerve pain—pain caused by
damage to the nerves from injury, sickle
cell blockage, or other conditions like diabetes. Nerve damage causes a burning, tingling, numbing
type of discomfort on a daily basis.

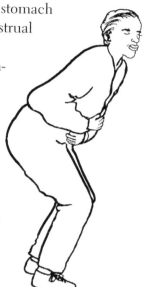

TREATING PAIN

1. Acute sickle cell pain episode. If this is a typical pain
episode, note the type of pain, then start by drinking more water,
lying down, and resting. Taking a warm bath can help, and so can
distractions, such as music, TV, a game, or relaxation techniques.
Massage to the area may be helpful. Or try moist heat (from a towel
placed in warm water then wrung out).

If your health care provider has given you pain medication,
start taking it as prescribed. Pain medications available without
prescription are:

Acetaminophen (one trade name is Tylenol). Acetaminophen
will block fever, so do not use it until a health care provider has
evaluated the fever and given the go ahead. Fever could mean a
serious life-threatening infection is present. Acetaminophen is

often combined with mild opiates like codeine (Tylenol #3) or hydrocodone (Vicoden). Be aware that these combinations will also block fever.

Ibuprofen (Motrin, Advil). Ibuprofen blocks pain in the muscles and bones. It does not cause drowsiness. Again, it can block fever, so it must not be used until the fever is evaluated. Ibuprofen can cause stomach upset and ulcers. It is best taken after a meal or snack. It can interfere with the ability of platelets to stop bleeding from cuts. Ibuprofen should not be used if there are kidney problems, stomach ulcers, bleeding problems, or asthma. This medication is good for menstrual cramps.

Aspirin. It has the same cautions as ibuprofen. One particular caution to note is that *aspirin has been associated with Reye's Syndrome and should not be given to children with fever or cold symptoms.*

Codeine and hydrocodone are milder opiate medications that block pain in the brain. These medications are usually given in combination with acetaminophen or ibuprofen but can be given by themselves to block pain when a fever is being monitored. They will not block fever, platelets, or cause stomach ulcers. These medications may cause drowsiness, nausea and itching. They are available by prescription only.

2. Acute pain from another cause. Pain in the head, chest, or abdomen and pain with fever should be evaluated, then the pain can be safely managed.

3. Chronic pain from sickle cell bone damage. The best treatment for this type of pain is long acting. Strategies include physical therapy, weight loss, carrying less weight, transcutaneous nerve stimulators (TNS), and mild heat. Long-acting arthritis medications are very helpful for daily pain control. The best medications for long pain relief, with the least side effects are the arthritis medications called non steroidal anti-inflammatory drugs, or NSAIDs for short. These include:

Pain Medications Available Without Prescription"

Name	Dosage by weight	Notes
Acetaminophen Tylenol	20 lbs—100mg 30 lbs—150mg 40 lbs—200mg 50 lbs—250 mg 60 lbs—300mg 70 lbs—350mg 80 lbs—400mg 90 lbs—450mg 100lbs– 500mg 120+—650mg	Use every 4 hours Will block fever Will not upset stomach Does not block inflammation Maximum Adult dose 4000mg /24hrs Toxic doses damage the liver
Ibuprofen Advil Motrin	20 lbs—100mg 30 lbs—150mg 40 lbs—200mg 50 lbs—250 mg 60 lbs—300mg 70 lbs—350mg 80 lbs—400mg 90 lbs—450mg 100lbs—500mg 120+—600mg	Give every 6 to 8 hours Will block a fever May cause stomach ulcers May damage kidneys May increase bleeding Does block inflammation Maximum adult dose 3200mg/24hr
Aspirin	Adults only 625 mg every 4–6 hours 80mg per day to slow clotting down.	All of the same notes as ibuprofen May cause Reye's Syndrome in children—do not use in children.

Salsalate (Disalcid), *Rofecoxib* (Vioxx), and *Celecoxib* (Celebrex). For long term use. Rofecoxib and Celecoxib are safer for the stomach than are other arthritis medications because they're associated with fewer stomach ulcers. Neither medication should be used if there are kidney problems.

Opioid medications may be used with the NSAIDs if the pain is not controlled, or alone if the NSAIDs cannot be used. The long acting opiates are morphine (MS Contin), oxycodone (Oxycontin) or methadone. All of these agents block pain in the brain and cause drowsiness, constipation, tolerance problems, physical dependence, and physical withdrawal if they are suddenly stopped. Antidepressant medications used along with the pain medication help fight chronic pain. A stool softener to prevent constipation should be used when opiates are being taken daily.

4. Chronic pain from other causes. All of the previous therapies listed are used to control chronic pain as are nerve blocks and disease-specific medications.

5. Chronic nerve pain or neuropathic pain. Treatment with anti-seizure medication has been helpful in pain control. One such medication is gabapentin (Neurontin).

IN THE EMERGENCY ROOM (ER)

The emergency room (ER) is the next stop if home treatment fails or if there is a danger sign such as

- fever
- weakness
- atypical pain
- headache
- chest pain
- abdominal pain

There are special emergency rooms for sickle cell patients in Atlanta and New York City. At present, most sickle cell patients must seek out the emergency room with the best possible care. Some hospitals may not have staff who are well trained in the care of sickle cell patients. The best defense is a good offense—come prepared with knowledge.

WHAT SHOULD HAPPEN

Here, in a nutshell, is what you should expect when you go into an emergency room:

- First your vital signs should be taken, including your temperature (normal 37.8°c or below), breathing rate (normal 15—20 per minute), heart rate—pulse (normal 80—100 per minute), blood pressure (normal 129/80), pulse oximetry, a measure of the oxygen in your red blood cells (normal 95% to 100%), and your pain intensity score (how much pain you are having from 0 to 10).

- A nurse should ask you about your main problem and assess how quickly you will be seen. In all ERs the most critical conditions must be seen first. A pain episode is not life-threatening, but there are symptoms that could require immediate treatment, such as fever, chills, headache, chest pain, abdominal pain, weakness, and abdominal swelling.

- A doctor, physician assistant, or nurse practitioner should examine you for signs of infection or complications. They should look in your ears, eyes, mouth, nose, and listen to your heart, chest and abdomen. They should also feel your abdomen for tenderness or swelling of the liver or spleen. They should check all of the areas that are hurting for swelling, heat, or tenderness.

- Blood tests, including a complete blood count (CBC), reticulocyte count and chemistry values may be done. A urine sample may be checked for blood, protein and infection.

- Your doctor may have developed an individual treatment plan for you. Generally, an IV or intravenous line should be started with D5W sugar (dextrose) in water to rehydrate the sickle red blood cells. Generally, normal saline should not be used.

- Pain medication should be given through the IV if possible, and on a fixed time schedule based on the medication. Giving medication on a fixed schedule assures a good pain-fighting blood level can be reached and kept. If pain medication is given as needed or as requested, the pain relief is like a roller coaster up and down. Pain medication given by Patient Controlled Analgesia or PCA pump allows a continuous amount to go in all the time. You can use the pump button to give extra doses at a safe rate for extra pain control. Your pain should be reassessed periodically to see if the medication is working.

- Try to continue distraction therapy by reading a book, watching TV, listening to music, or playing a game. Relaxation techniques can be used.

COMMON MEDICATIONS USED IN ER'S

Many good pain medications are available for pain episodes and many work better in combinations. Among those frequently used are:

- Morphine. Morphine is an opiate that blocks pain in the brain. It can be given by mouth, IV, in a patient-controlled analgesia pump (PCA), or by a shot in the muscle. Morphine takes effect in fifteen minutes and lasts up to three hours. It slows breathing down as the dose goes up. It can cause itching, nausea, vomiting, and constipation. The body can become physically dependent on morphine for several days after use. In coming off of morphine, the dose should be tapered off and not stopped suddenly.

- Nalbuphine (Nubain). Nalbuphine is an injectable pain medication that is safe and effective in controlled doses. It does not slow respiration as morphine does. Nalbuphine has a "ceiling effect," so if it does not control pain as required, you must switch to another medication. This medication has fewer side effects with less itching, nausea, and drowsiness than morphine. Nalbuphine may cause withdrawal symptoms in patients taking daily opiates (MS Contin, Oxycontin, Methadone, and others) and it should not be used in those patients. Nalbuphine is a great first choice for those not on chronic opiates.

- Ketorolac (Toradol). This is an IV, non-steroidal anti-inflammatory drug that blocks pain in the bone and muscle tissue where the blocked blood flow from sickled red cells has caused damage. All of the cautions are the same as for ibuprofen. This medication can only be used for a maximum of five days continuously.
- Meperidine (Demerol). This opiate pain medication is good for acute pain, but not for pain lasting more than a few days. It breaks down in the body to a substance that can cause seizures in high doses. This medication has all of the same cautions as morphine, which is a better first choice opiate.
- Hydroxyzine (Vistaril). In proper doses, Hydroxyzine can prevent nausea and itching caused by opiates. It can also help calm fear.

ADDICTION TO OPIATES

All opiate medications can cause the body to become dependant upon them after several days of continuous use. This is called physical dependence. The body then requires higher doses of the opiate to get adequate pain control. This is called tolerance.

If any of the opiate medications are used for several days and then withdrawn, the body will have withdrawal symptoms such as cramps, sweating, abdominal pain and shakes.

Withdrawal can be avoided by slowly decreasing the amount of the medication used over several days to allow the body to adjust.

True drug addiction occurs in 5% to 10% of patients on daily opiates. At the Georgia Comprehensive Sickle Cell Center, we followed over 2400 sickle cell patients and only 5% met the standard for drug addiction.

There is also a condition we call "pseudo-addiction." Patients who have been undertreated with opiates may experience uncontrolled pain and withdrawal symptoms. Some—indeed, too many—health care workers mislabel these patients as "addicts with drug-seeking behavior."

Until more sickle cell centers are available, patients with pain must keep returning to the ER for help. A good understanding of how opiates work and the proper doses of long-acting medications can stop this vicious cycle.

ADMISSION TO THE HOSPITAL

Admission to the hospital is recommended under the following conditions:

- for pain management or treatment, especially if the pain does not go down to a manageable level after 8–12 hours of treatment in the ER or if a complication is present. A complication is present under these circumstances:
  — You need to return for more therapy within 48 hours of previous inpatient or outpatient treatment of a pain episode.
  — You are experiencing a pain episode, along with any of the following:
  — infection
  — temperature over 38° C
  — pneumonia
  — kidney infection
  — blood infection (sepsis)
  — low blood oxygen or too much acid in the blood
  — stroke

— pregnancy
— heart problems or failure
— priapism that will not go away
— blood clots in the lung
— decrease in blood counts
— liver inflammation, gallstones, or gall bladder inflammation

AS AN INPATIENT

After you are admitted into the hospital, treatment started in the ER should continue. There are several things you can do to ensure adequate pain management:

- Let the staff know your pain intensity level as a number from 0 to 10.
- Tell the nurses if you are having side effects like nausea, vomiting, constipation, itching, or feeling drowsy.
- Report your mood to the nursing staff. Feelings of depression, fear, anger, and sadness can all hinder your pain treatment. Counsel from chaplains, social workers, nurses, as well as medication, can help in many cases.

Medication by Patient Controlled Analgesia (PCA) pump is one of the best options for pain control in the hospital. Report to your nurse any change in symptoms, or sites of pain.

RELAXATION TECHNIQUES

Pain can be helped by thinking about something else. Dwelling on the pain can make it feel worse. Being tense tightens muscles, reduces blood flow and increases pain. Relaxation techniques help you relax muscles and get your mind off of the pain.

Start by getting in a quiet room, with some soothing music if it is available. Get in a comfortable position. Make a fist, release your fingers and concentrate on letting them go limp. Tense your arm muscles and then let them go limp. Tense your shoulders, then let them go limp. Tense your neck then let it go limp. "Squench" your face muscles and let them go limp. Tense your toes and feet, then let them go limp. Tense your leg muscles, and let them go limp. Tense your stomach and let it go limp.

At this stage, all of your muscles should be more relaxed. If any feel tense, repeat, tightening and letting the tense muscles go until they are relaxed. Think of a calm place that you have visited like a beach or park. Meditate on your favorite scriptures, song or event. Biofeedback can help train you to relax.

CONCLUSION

Discuss your pain management plan with your health care provider when you are well and not in pain. Make a plan that is right for you. Keep this plan with you, after filling in the important information to share with each health care provider you see.

There are free, problem oriented guidelines for sickle syndromes available for health care providers on the internet twenty-four hours a day at the Sickle Cell Information Center at http://www.emory.edu/PEDS/SICKLE.

CHAPTER 15

New Treatments and Research

J ust beyond today's effective treatments are a second line of
treatments, still being tested and refined. Patients involved in
these new treatments hold a special place in the list of sickle
cell heroines and heroes.

KEON'S STORY

Keon Penn underwent the world's first unrelated stem cell transplant at Egelston Children's Hospital in Atlanta on December 11,
1998. Keon had been receiving monthly blood transfusions at
Grady ever since he had a stroke at age five. He had been coming
regularly to the hospital ever since. Now, at the age of twelve, Keon
had become a pioneer.

Currently, the only methods of preventing future strokes is lifelong, monthly blood transfusions or a bone marrow transplant that
completely replaces the patient's blood- making factory with donor
cells.

Keon did not have a brother or sister match to donate non-
sickle cell bone marrow, so the next logical step was to use stem
cells from umbilical cord blood from an unrelated donor. Stem
cells are very early cells that can produce blood cells when placed
in the bone marrow. Keon was the first to open the door for many

sickle cell patients who do not have a close match but who have enough complications to merit the risk of the procedure.

Two years after the transplant, Keon is free of sickle cell but is still battling his body's attempts to reject the donor stem cells. Keon and his family are brave pioneers in the quest for a cure that will some day be available to all of those with sickle cell disease.

TRANSPLANTS: A PROBLEMATIC CURE

In addition to the treatments discussed, a cure for sickle cell anemia already actually exists. That cure is bone marrow transplantation. You might wonder why, if there is a cure, doctors still treat the disease with potentially dangerous drugs that do not cure.

There are two good answers to that. First, suitable bone marrow donors are not easy to come by. Second, bone marrow transplantation is itself a risky proposition. The short and intermediate term risks of recipient death are 5 percent and 10 percent respectively, and there is also risk of serious infections, graft rejection, and graft versus host disease.

Furthermore, the donor runs the risk of anesthesia damage, and, rarely, infection; these are much smaller, but still real, risks.

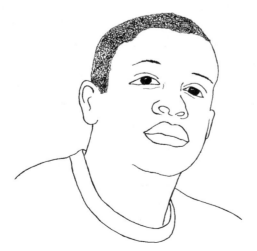

The high cost of bone marrow transplantation and follow-up care must also be considered. It's obvious that this procedure is not a leisurely stroll through the park.

MATCHING TISSUE TYPES

Different blood types or red blood cell incompatibility is not a barrier to successful bone marrow transplantation (as it is for blood transfusion). But donor and recipient must be closely matched in tissue type, also referred to as HLA type. In general, the closer the two tissue types resemble each other, the better the chance of a successful transplantation.

Several sophisticated techniques are available for determining the tissue type of donor and recipient.

For most patients an HLA matched brother or sister, if available, is the best choice as a bone marrow donor. In general, *any two siblings have about one chance in four of sharing the same HLA type.*

In relation to sickle cell anemia itself, the same genetic laws dictate that if both parents each carry one sickle trait (allele), one out of four of their children will have the sickle cell disease, and two of every four would inherit the sickle trait. If we choose only siblings who, in addition to sharing the same HLA, have neither sickle cell disease nor sickle trait, then the chance of finding a suitable donor among one's brothers and sisters shrinks to about 7.5 percent.

Because of the difficulty of finding an unaffected, HLA-compatible donor among one's own siblings, sometimes another family member, or an unrelated person who is HLA compatible, can donate bone marrow instead.

Although unrelated bone marrow transplants have a higher failure rate than transplants between completely matched siblings, they also are often successful.

The National Marrow Donor Program has been developed to assist in the search for compatible donors in the United States. Its toll-free telephone numbers are 1-800-573-6667 and 1-800-526-7809. Its website is www.marrow.org.

QUALIFYING FOR BONE MARROW TRANSPLANTATION

Bone marrow transplants are not given lightly. In order to qualify for one, the patient, with the help of the his doctor and family, must do a great deal of preparation:

1. Sickle cell eligibility. Whether the transplantation is appropriate to consider depends on whether your child has had severe enough sickle cell disease to make the risks of bone marrow transplant worthwhile. To help the appraisal, patients should provide a summary of their medical history. The summary should focus on whether the child has had stroke and chronic transfusion, frequent hospital stays for pain or lung problems, or other major sickle cell problems. This information can be provided by fax or e-mail.
2. Other medical issues. Make your doctor aware that your family is considering the bone marrow transplant (BMT) option. Ask the doctor to let the potential transplant team know if there are any hidden medical problems that might influence your decision, such as chronic viral or other infections, problems with transfusion reactions, other medical problems unrelated to sickle cell, or anything else unusual. At this point the statement doesn't have to be lengthy or formal. It is more like a safety check to make sure that the potential transplant team doesn't miss any significant medical issues. A more complete medical record will be required later.
3. HAL-typing blood tests. Do HLA typing of your child and the relative with the highest probability of matching. Only brothers or sisters from the same parents are really potential donors. Parents and half-siblings are unlikely to match unless there

was an unusual family tree. If the sibling is not a full HLA match, then it is very unlikely that BMT can be done. HLA typing will cost several thousand dollars.

4. Pre-BMT evaluation. After all of the above steps, a formal evaluation by the BMT team can begin. This will include a detailed look at the child's medical history and current medical condition, plus a look at the family's ability to cope with the difficult BMT process. Parents will need to stay with the patient for a minimum of 8 months for the pre-transplant evaluation, transplant stay, and post-transplant follow-up. A financial arrangement will need to be made, since the cost for the BMT process can run from $150,000 to $250,000. An outside expert panel will review the case on ethical grounds.

5. BMT and early follow-up period. The overall success rate of BMT as a cure for sickle cell disease is 80% to 85%, but bone marrow transplant is a risky process, with a 5% to 8% chance of death. Death can be caused by infection, bleeding, toxic effects of the treatment, or the new bone marrow engrafting and then attacking the rest of the body. There is also a 10% to 12% chance that the child could go through the BMT process but reject the new bone marrow, ending up still having sickle cell disease.

This procedure requires close medical follow up. It also means taking many medications daily.

THE TRANSPLANTATION PROCESS

Bone marrow transplantation can be understood by dividing the process into three phases:

- preparation for transplantation
- transplantation
- post-transplantation management

Preparing for Transplantation

Before transplantation, high dose chemotherapy, sometimes with radiation therapy, is given to the person receiving the bone marrow (host). The purpose is to destroy the host's immune system to prevent rejection of the bone marrow graft. Chemotherapy, and possibly radiation treatments, remove the old blood-making factory so the new transplanted one can take over.

The use of chemotherapy drugs, singly or in combination, is challenging because they can be toxic to organ systems other than the bone marrow. Further, the combination of chemotherapy plus radiotherapy may not completely kill all the host's bone marrow cells, even though it may damage other vulnerable organ systems.

Transplantation

Donor bone marrow is usually taken from the large pelvic bones, but it may also be obtained from the breast bone, ribs, or (in children), the large bone of the lower leg. The donor bone marrow is sucked out (doctors call this *aspiration*) with a special needle and syringe under general anesthesia, with the donor asleep, or spinal anesthesia, with the donor awake.

The bone marrow suspension is then given to the recipient intravenously. *The bone marrow stem cells* (the immature cells that will develop into the mature blood cell types) pass through the recipient's lungs and find their way to the bone marrow cavities, where they will grow and mature if all goes well.

Generally, two to four weeks are needed following transplantation before the transplanted marrow can produce enough mature red and white blood cells and platelets to sustain a healthy system.

Post-transplantation Management

During the two to four weeks following transplantation, the patient needs to be isolated to protect against infection that can be life-threatening. Both bacterial and fungal infections can occur, but the infections can be treated with antibiotic and anti-fungal drugs.

Platelet transfusions may be necessary during this period to prevent serious bleeding. Transfusions of special white blood cells (*granulocytes*) may be required to combat serious infections.

Packed red blood cells may also be transfused as needed to prevent symptoms of anemia, although those with sickle cell diseases are often better adapted to withstand anemia (because of their chronic anemia) than are most other recipients of bone marrow transplants.

Nourishment

Patients coming to bone marrow transplantation are often poorly nourished as a result of their disease. Also, chemotherapy and radiation treatments before the transplant often cause decreased appetite, nausea, and/or vomiting, which may make eating and drinking uncomfortable or even painful. These treatments may also interfere with stomach function and with the intestinal absorption of nutrients. Patients routinely require intravenous feeding.

Successful Transplantation

The average time needed for successful bone transplantation is up to six months including preparation, the transplant, recovery, and intensive follow-up. Doctors determine the success of the transplant by blood and genetic tests.

Complications

Complications may follow even successful bone marrow transplantation. Such complications are:

- graft rejection (a more common problem in people with aplastic anemia)
- infection
- acute graft versus host disease (GVHD)
- cardiomyopathy (a disorder of the heart muscle)
- cataracts (a clouding of the lens of the eye resulting in visual impairment)
- liver problems caused by blockage of liver veins

- leukoencephalopathy, a rare neurologic condition that occurs chiefly in people with weakened immune systems. It generally lasts from one to six months and almost spontaneous remissions (cures, either temporary or permanent) have been reported.

Marrow Graft Rejection

Marrow graft rejection occurs when the host's immune system has been so sensitized by blood transfusions that it is on a kind of hair trigger; or when the immune system hasn't been adequately suppressed with chemotherapy.

Bone marrow graft failure may also occur for reasons that have nothing to do with the immune system, such as too few donor cells getting into the recipient, or if there's something wrong in the environment of the bone marrow cavity that prevents the transplanted stem cells from thriving.

Acute Graft Versus Host Disease

Acute graft versus host disease (GVHD) happens when transplanted white blood cells fight against the host's tissues. Even when the donor and the host are completely matched, there are usually minor differences between their cells. The risk to hosts of developing GVDH, even if the donor is a closely matched sibling, is 50 percent. Those who have had many blood transfusions before the transplant are at a higher risk for GVHD.

Acute GVHD usually involves the skin, the digestive system, and the liver. A skin rash is often the first sign. Diarrhea, abdominal pain, and intestinal paralysis may result from the intestinal involvement. Severe immunologic deficiency may develop with a risk of life-threatening infection.

GVHD can be prevented with powerful drugs, although these carry dangers of their own. In about two-thirds of the cases, acute GVHD can be treated successfully by using a type of antibody together with steroids or drugs that suppress the immune system.

Features of the chronic form of GVHD

- skin rashes
- inflammation of the corneas and conjunctivae (the outer lining of the corneas and the inner lining of the eyelids)
- inflammation of the mucous membranes of the mouth
- narrowing of the esophagus and inflammation of the intestines
- respiratory (lung) failure
- chronic liver damage
- wasting (loss of muscle, fat, and bone tissue)

Treating GVHD with prednisone (a steroid), sometimes in combination with a chemical agent that suppresses the immune system, results in recovery for about 80 percent of patients. However, treatment for one to three years is often required.

During these long periods of treatment, measures must be in place to prevent such steroid-associated complications as bone loss, kidney stones, muscle wasting, low potassium, and abnormalities of carbohydrate and fat metabolism such as diabetes. Steroids are strong and useful medicine, but they may cause secondary complications of their own.

The greatest threat to the host during chronic GVHD is opportunistic infections, that is, infections that take advantage of the patient's weakened condition. The timely use of antibiotics and other drugs may reduce both the frequency and severity of infections. By the end of the first year after transplantation, the immune systems of most recipients have recovered and the patients no longer experience frequent or severe infections.

Immunologic Tolerance

Researchers have much to learn about how to keep host cells from reacting against donor immune cells, but each day brings more knowledge. Some of what we do know is this:

- Younger patients reject donor bone marrow less commonly than older patients.
- Bone marrow transplantations on hosts who haven't received any blood transfusions have a higher success rate.
- Host obesity is a risk factor for poor transplantation outcome, so every effort must be made to achieve and maintain ideal body weight in obese patients.

Other Complications of Bone Marrow Transplantation

Other complications include:

- non-infectious pneumonia
- liver disease
- infertility
- sexual dysfunction
- delayed immune recovery

Venoocclusive Liver Disease

Venoocclusive liver disease, caused by drugs used in chemotherapy, occurs in about half of bone marrow transplant recipients. It causes blockage of veins in the liver, and its symptoms include:

- jaundice
- enlargement of the liver, which may become painful and tender to touch
- accumulation of fluid in the abdominal and pelvic cavities

With proper treatment, about 70 percent of patients ultimately recover from venoocclusive liver disease.

Hemolytic Uremic Syndrome or HUS

HUS is a kind of anemia that usually begins four to eight weeks after the last dose of a chemotherapeutic drug, but it may occur up to several months later. It is caused by the chemotherapy itself.

The symptoms of HUS include:

- shortness of breath
- weakness
- fatigue
- decreased urination
- spontaneous bruising
- high blood pressure
- filling up of the lungs with fluid
- abnormalities in the heart's rhythm
- inflammation of the membrane surrounding the heart
- accumulation of fluid between the heart and the membrane surrounding it

HUS is fatal in about 50 percent of cases.

THE FUTURE OF BONE MARROW TRANSPLANT

Research is now underway to see if it is safer to destroy part of the bone marrow producing sickle red blood cells before transplanting donor marrow. This would leave a mix of sickle and normal red cells, but the benefit from the normal cells. The question is whether the benefit from the normal cells is enough to prevent pain events and complications.

Another area of research centers on doing a bone marrow transplant to the baby with sickle cell disease while it is in the mother's womb. This would be less costly and the mother's womb would serve as the recovery area.

Scientists have also been able to use their genetic knowledge to alter genes and breed mice with sickle cell hemoglobin. This allows researchers to test new medications and treatments without any harm to people.

Follow the research news at the sickle cell information web site for updates.

AGENTS TO BLOCK PLATELETS

The Comprehensive Sickle Cell Center in Atlanta is studying whether or not N3 fatty acids (fish oil) reduce coagulation in sickle cell patients. Those treated for one year with the N3 fatty acids had half as many pain events as did the patients who received a placebo. A multicenter trial is in progress to determine the efficacy of this treatment to prevent pain episodes and sickle complications.

HYDROXUREA AND HEMOGLOBIN F

Between conception and birth our predominant hemoglobin is hemoglobin F (fetal hemoglobin). Having a high percentage of circulating hemoglobin as hemoglobin F protects against sickling and its many complications. We know this because infants with sickle cell disease do not usually have apparent problems until after about six months of age, when the levels of hemoglobin F have fallen substantially. Also, those with sickle cell diseases of Shi ancestry from Saudi Arabia, and patients from certain parts of India who have high levels of hemoglobin F, seem to get milder versions of the disease.

In short, a high percentage of hemoglobin F in a patient with sickle cell disease means that the patient is less likely to suffer complications.

The drug hydroxyurea in combination with erythropoietin, has proven effective in raising the percentage of hemoglobin F by stimulating the production of protective fetal hemoglobin within the red cells.

Adult patients on hydroxyurea have 50 percent fewer pain

episodes, 50 percent fewer blood transfusions and 50 percent less need for hospitalization. Studies in children have shown efficacy and short term safety, but the long term effects are unknown.

The benefits of hydroxyurea are:

- decreased frequency and severity of pain crises
- decreased frequency and severity of acute chest syndrome
- decreased need for blood transfusions

But there are also problems and restrictions to its use. Because hydroxyurea, like other strong medications, has potential side effects, its use is reserved for the most severely ill sickle cell patients. *Its safety for use in children with sickle cell anemia is not yet supported by any studies.*

All available brands of hydroxyurea contain some lactose as a filler. About 70 percent of African Americans and a similar percentage of other groups prone to sickle cell anemia are lactose intolerant after childhood. Reactions may include,

- bloating
- increased intestinal gas
- diarrhea and nausea

Because hydroxyurea may harm or destroy an unborn baby, *a woman of child-bearing age must use a very reliable means of birth control while taking this drug.* If she is planning a pregnancy, she must stop taking this drug several months before attempting conception.

Because hydroxyurea is present in the breast milk of women taking the drug, *nursing women should avoid using it.*

And because hydroxyurea may also cause genetic changes in developing sperm cells and a decrease in the sperm count, *men should not take hydroxyurea for at least three months before attempting conception with their partners.*

Apart from the possible side effects already discussed, other rare but serious side effects of hydroxyurea, such as leukemia and skin cancer, can occur. Less severe, but more frequent side effects reported in people taking hydroxyurea include

- bleeding not due to low platelet counts
- an increased frequency of infection
- gastrointestinal disturbances
- rashes
- weight gain
- hair loss
- darkening of toenails and fingernails

Hydroxyurea should not be used

- if your total white blood cell count is less than 2,500 because this could seriously reduce your ability to resist infection
- if your platelet count is below 100,000, because this could increase your risk of serious bleeding
- if you have severe anemia, because your red blood cell count and hemoglobin could fall too low and your vital organs not receive enough oxygen.

LABORATORY TESTS YOU SHOULD HAVE BEFORE STARTING HYDROXYUREA

Before starting hydroxyurea patients should have the following laboratory tests done:

- a complete blood count, which includes hemoglobin, hematocrit, white blood cells, and platelets
- liver function and kidney function tests

These tests need to be repeated frequently during therapy.

Patients taking hydroxyurea most often have to stop the drug to allow their low cell counts to come back up to a safe level (which usually occurs within two weeks of stopping).

MONITORING HYDROXYUREA

Complete blood counts must be done at least every two weeks while the patient is taking hydroxyurea. If the counts remain in an acceptable range, then the dose may be increased every twelve weeks over twenty-four consecutive weeks until the highest tolerated dose (35 mg/kg/day) is reached.

HYDROXYUREA FOR PATIENTS WITH IMPAIRED KIDNEY FUNCTION

Since hydroxyurea is mostly eliminated from the body by the kidneys, the dosage often has to be reduced in patients with impaired kidney function—unfortunately, a fairly common situation in patients with sickle cell disease.

ERYTHROPOIETIN IN COMBINATION WITH HYRDROXYUREA

The hormone erythropoietin (Epogen or Procrit) may increase the effectiveness, and reduce the risk, of treatment with hydroxyurea.

AGENTS TO HELP RED CELLS FLOW BETTER

Inhaled, nitric oxide (NO) is a gas that, even in small amounts, causes smooth muscle in the blood vessel wall to relax and the entire vessel to dilate. In tests, even at the lowest concentrations, NO slowed cell sickling and even promoted the unsickling of sickled cells. The higher the concentration of NO, the stronger the favorable effect. Current studies are testing the effect of inhaled NO on the length and severity of acute pain episodes.

CPC-111 appears to reduce the red blood cell sickling that causes the blood starvation-induced tissue damage in sickle cell pain episode. Patients treated with this drug had significantly lower pain scores (on two different scales) than placebo-treated patients. Phase III trials are underway in patients with sickle pain episodes.

RheothRx (Flocor) is an intravascular agent. By essentially creating a coating on the damaged cells, Flocor is designed to allow blood cells to "slip over" one another, improving blood flow and restoring oxygen delivery, according to the manufacturer. Flocor is now in a phase III trial for sickle cell patients suffering from vascular occlusive pain episode.

Trental (a generic name for pentoxifylline) belongs to a group of drugs such as:

- caffeine
- theophylline, a stimulant found in tea and used in the treatment of asthma and bronchitis
- theobromine, the main stimulant found in chocolate

This drug is known to have several actions that are potentially helpful in sickle cell disease. Trental

- increases the production of a molecule that helps the red blood cells keep their flexibility and not break down and grow stiff
- lowers blood fibrinogen levels and thus cuts down on clogging
- improves blood flow in other ways

Not all patients are able to tolerate Trental. It is certainly much safer than hydroxyurea or bone marrow transplantation, but we don't know much yet about how safe it is for young children, for pregnant women, or for nursing mothers and their infants.

A small percentage of patients taking Trental experience digestive side effects and a slightly increased tendency to bleed. Other people taking Trental may experience palpitations (rapid, irregular, or unusually forceful heartbeats), tremor, insomnia, or nervousness. In other words, the side effects are similar to those that some people get from coffee.

AGENTS THAT INCREASE RED CELL WATER

Keeping the red blood cell full of water prevents the sickle hemoglobin from deforming. Clotrimazole, an oral antifungal that blocks the loss of potassium from the red blood cell, prevents the increase in sickle cell hemoglobin concentration and reduces sickling.

SECOND CONDITIONS THAT INCREASE BLOOD VISCOSITY

The last subject we want to talk about in this chapter is how other conditions, in addition to sickle cell disease itself, can increase the stickiness of the blood. In most cases people with sickle cell trait do not have symptoms unless they are exposed to very high altitudes or to dehydration.

But there are exceptions to this general rule peculiar to patients who, in addition to sickle cell trait, have a second condition which increases the blood's viscosity or stickiness.

One such condition is rheumatoid arthritis, in which the tendency of the platelets to stick to one another, and possibly to the red blood cells, is increased. Other conditions characterized by increased blood viscosity include diabetes mellitus. It is also possible that people with sickle cell trait and diabetes may be more susceptible to the small vessel complications of diabetes, which include disorders of the back of the eye, of the kidneys, and of the heart.

GENE THERAPY

Researchers at Duke University Medical Center have shown that they can use a new type of gene therapy to correct the sickle cell hemoglobin defect in human blood cells. The results of their laboratory studies, published in the June 5, 1998, issue of the journal

Science, show that successful gene therapy may lie not in correcting faulty DNA, the storehouse of genetic information, but in correcting the RNA, which translates that genetic information to the protein synthesis machinery of a cell. The researchers plan to begin testing the therapy in sickle cell patients within a few years.

CHAPTER 16

What You Can Do

THE POWER OF ONE

Twenty-five years ago in Atlanta, when her son Carey was eight, doctors told Berrutha Harper that her son would die before his teen years of sickle cell disease. Berrutha had to take her son to the local emergency rooms for pain treatment, and she often experienced long waits and had to deal with health care providers who had little or no sickle cell experience.

When Berrutha saw that she couldn't get consistently good care in ordinary emergency rooms, she began to dream of an emergency room dedicated to the needs of sickle cell patients, with a specially trained staff of health care providers who would treat patients with knowledge and compassion.

Berrutha was the kind of dreamer who saw a dream as possibility. She organized other parents and patients into a group of people who could share their concerns about sickle cell patients and consider how to improve sickle cell care in the largest of the Atlanta hospitals, Grady Memorial.

The hospital received many patient complaints each day about the care given to emergency room sickle cell patients. But the hospital's official position was that it couldn't afford an emergency room dedicated exclusively to the treatment of sickle cell patients.

Berrutha was not the kind of woman to give up easily. She set out to get state funding from the legislature. During lunch breaks from her job as a medical clerk in a local health care clinic, she would go to the state capitol building and knock on legislators' doors.

One day, a patient came into the emergency room with chest pain, and was treated for sickle cell pain crisis. The patient died of a heart attack, a diagnosis not thought of because the patient had sickle cell disease. Berrutha called all of the parent/patient groups to stage a protest march in front of the state capitol. Berrutha arrived at the capitol with signs in hand, but no people showed up to march. A discouraged Berrutha sat on the steps and sent up a short prayer. A group of school bus drivers from south Georgia, who had delivered a group of school children for a capitol tour, asked Berrutha about the protest signs and got an education about sickle cell disease. The bus drivers asked if they could carry the signs for Berrutha, since they were waiting for the school kids to return. The news of the marching bus drivers reached the inner chambers of the legislators in session. The leader of the Black Caucus came outside and invited Berrutha to meet with him if she would call off the march. This was the first time Berrutha's story was heard by the influential leaders of the legislature. Funds were allocated to Grady Memorial Hospital to start a twenty-four hour clinic with a dedicated staff of health care providers trained to care for sickle cell patients.

In September, 1984, the Sickle Cell Center opened its doors for patients. It has been open ever since, providing round the clock emergency care, comprehensive preventive care, research, inpatient consultations and education. All of this was the result of one mother's prayer, vision, and perseverance.

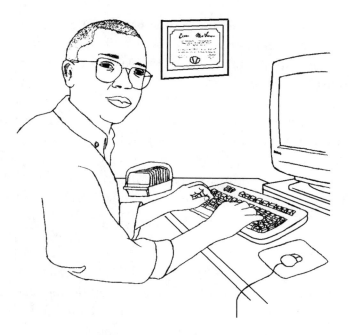

FUND RAISING

There are several ways to raise money for your sickle cell activities. First set up or partner with a 501C3 tax exempt organization so donations can be tax deductible. Many hospitals, church and civic groups have this status. Plan a budget. Funds will be needed for scholarships for college, emergency needs of patients, research projects and education. Fund raising activities include walk-a-thons, bowl-a-thons, banquets, and concerts. Invite corporate participation and invite the local press to do a story on the event. This will raise awareness about sickle cell disease and raise funds at the same time.

BLOOD DRIVES

It is important to reduce the formation of antibodies in sickle cell patients. The best way to do this is to transfuse blood from people of the same ethnic background. If sickle cell disease primarily effects those in the African American community in your area, then blood donations should be increased in that community to reduce the antigen exposure. The more antibodies a patient makes, the more difficult it is to find blood that matches and will not cause a transfusion reaction.

Get involved by organizing a blood drive in your civic or church group. Contact the local Red Cross chapter which can help you set up a blood drive. Ask about a "Partner for Life" program, in which a group of donors can be matched to a specific sickle cell patient to reduce the blood exposure and reduce the making of antibodies. At the blood drives, educate the public about sickle cell disease and the need for regular blood donations.

HEALTH FAIRS

Health fairs are good places to educate the public about sickle cell disease. Set up a table with informational handouts and have people on hand to answer questions. If possible, provide sickle cell screening by drawing blood for hemoglobin electrophoresis. You can network with other community based health organizations to help support sickle cell patients.

PUBLIC EDUCATION

Educate the public in your community by inviting the local newspaper and TV news to do stories about patients and events in your area. Sickle cell patients have wonderfully inspirational life stories of overcoming pain and hardship. Talk about innovative support groups or new advances in research.

POLITICS

Tell your legislators about sickle cell disease and the need for services in your community. States can be involved in newborn screening, funding comprehensive centers, funding vocational rehabilitation programs and funding preventive care. You can contact legislators by newsletters, personal calls, personal visits, and e-mail. Invite them to your educational events. National leaders need to be educated about the unique needs of sickle cell patients and the need for increased research funding. Sickle cell is the most common genetic disease in the United States but it is underfunded compared to other less common genetic diseases such as hemophilia and cystic fibrosis.

SICKLE CELL CAMP

Many sickle cell centers and foundations in major cities have annual sickle cell summer camp for children. Camp is a way for children to interact with their peers in a fun environment. Usually medical support is provided by the medical teams from the sickle cell centers. Campers are encouraged to drink extra fluids, take rest breaks, and avoid high temperature exposure. Usually these camps charge a small fee to cover lodging and food. Frequently, scholarships are provided to those who do not have any resources. To locate a camp, contact the nearest sickle cell center or the Sickle Cell Disease Association of America for the chapter nearest to you.

SUPPORT GROUPS
WHY SUPPORT AND COUNSELING ARE VITAL

Sickle cell disease is not only an anemia of the blood. Like all serious illness it affects every aspect of the patient's life, and the physical ills can be made worse by intense emotional and social stress. Without proper medical attention and support from those organized to help, the psychological component of this disease can prove to be as devastating as the disease itself.

In some respects, better treatment and care of sickle cell patients have intensified the emotional and psychological problems associated with the disease. Because life expectancies have increased, patients can face a seemingly unending prospect of absence from school and work, poor employment prospects, and managed care crises. Depression, boredom, anti-social and self-destructive behavior are expressions of the intense emotional strain the patient faces daily.

The very good news is that sickle cell patients don't have to face the disease alone. From initial screening through every stage and pain episode, counseling and support is available. One only has to look.

Not only is immediate help available to the patient, but counseling and support are also there for family and friends, teachers, employers, and health care professionals. In fact, it is the interconnected efforts of the entire sickle cell community that is key to successful support.

What we offer you here, to start you on your journey, is a basic list of the resources that will get you started. Once you take the first step, you'll find that the appropriate path will be obvious. Simply walk it, as you do any walk, one step at a time.

What you will soon see is that each organization is a link in a long, interconnected chain of support, a chain that has grown much stronger in the past thirty years, as we have all come to better understand the needs of the sickle cell patient.

THE KINDS OF FACILITIES AVAILABLE

Once you start, you'll soon find that

- Some agencies are government sponsored but many are community based
- Some focus on education and clinical research for the medical community
- Some stress political activism in their efforts to generate the funds for clinical research and community outreach programs

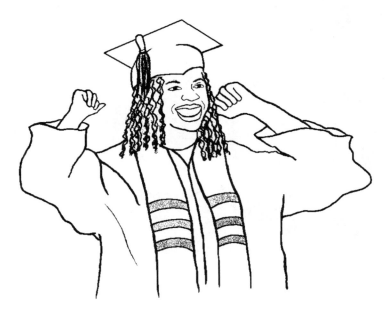

- Others stress the one-on-one of personal involvement and individual care

Whatever the approach, their goal is the same—to fight for the health and rights of the individual sickle cell patient.

CHAPTER 17

Resources

NATIONAL ORGANIZATIONS
COMPREHENSIVE SICKLE CELL CENTERS:
THE GOVERNMENT'S ROLE

In 1972, in a key step toward greater sickle cell disease awareness, the National Institutes of Health (NIH) created Comprehensive Sickle Cell Centers (CSCCs). Although their main emphasis is clinical research, the CSCCs provide community services such as screening, counseling and education.

Here is a list of the Comprehensive Sickle Cell Centers as of September 2001. These may change every five years because of the federal government's funding cycles. (You may find the list and other useful information on the new NIH sickle cell center's website: www.rhofed.com/sickle.) These centers form a national framework within which many other support resources are linked across the nation and around the world.

Johnson Haynes, Jr., M.D.
Director, Comprehensive Sickle Cell Center
University of South Alabama Comprehensive Sickle Cell Center
307 University Blvd.
CSAB 223
Mobile, AL 36688

334-460-7334
334-460-6604
kbilling@usamail.usouthal.edu

Ronald W. Helms, Ph.D.
Director, Statistics and Management Center
Rho Federal Systems Divisions, Inc.
100 Eastowne Dr.
Chapel Hill, NC 27514
919-408-8000 ext. 222
919-408-0999
RonHelms_CSCC@rhoworld.com

Cage S. Johnson, M.D.
Director, Comprehensive Sickle Cell Center
University of Southern California
Department of Medicine
RMR 304
2025 Zonal Avenue
Los Angeles, CA 90033
cagejohn@hsc.usc.edu

Clinton H. Joiner, M.D., Ph.D.
Director, Cincinnati Comprehensive Sickle Cell Center
Children's Hospital Medical Center
Division of Hematology/Oncology
3333 Burnet Avenue
Cincinnati, OH 45229-3039
513-636-4541
513-636-5562
clintjoiner@chmcc.org

Martin Steinberg, M.D.
Director, Comprehensive Sickle Cell Center

Boston Medical Center
One Boston Medical Center Place, FGH-2
Boston, MA 02118
617-414-1020
617-414-1021
lmcmahon@bu.edu

William C. Mentzer
Director, Northern California Comprehensive Sickle Cell Center
San Francisco General Hospital
Building 100, Room 331
1001 Potrero Avenue
San Francisco, CA 94110
415-206-5169
415-206-3071
wmentzner@fghpeds.ucsf.edu

Ronald L. Nagel, M. D.
Director, Bronx Comprehensive Sickle Cell Center
Albert Einstein College of Medicine
Division of Hematology
Ullman Building, Room 921
1300 Morris Park Avenue
Bronx, NY 10461
718-430-2088
718-824-3153
nagel@accom.yu.edu

Kwaku Ohene-Frempong, M.D.
Director, Comprehensive Sickle Cell Center
The Children's Hospital of Philadelphia
34th Street & Civic Center Blvd.
Philadelphia, PA 19104
215-590-3423

215-590-2499
ohene-frempong@email.chop.edu

Sergio Piomelli, M.D.
Director, Comprehensive Sickle Cell Center of Manhattan
Columbia University
College of Physicians and Surgeons
630 West 168th Street
New York, NY 10032
212-305-6531
212-305-8408
sp23@columbia.edu

Tim M. Townes, Ph.D.
Director, Comprehensive Sickle Cell Center
Univ. of Alabama-Birmingham
UAB Station THT-513-A
Birmingham, AL 35924-0006
Phone: 205-975-2280
Fax: 205-975-5264
eskridge@uab.deu

Marie J. Stuart, M.D.
Director, Marian Anderson Sickle Cell Anemia Care and
    Research Center
Thomas Jefferson University
Division of Hematology
Department of Pediatrics
College Bldg., Suite 727
1025 Walnut Street
Philadelphia, PA 19107
215-955-9820
215-955-8011
marie.stuart@mail.tju.edu

KEY COMMUNITY ORGANIZATIONS ON THE WEB

The worldwide web is an invaluable resource for researching sickle cell support groups. Key organizations, such as the American Sickle Cell Anemia Association (ASCAA), the Sickle Cell Disease Association of America (SCDAA), and Sickle Cell Advocates for Research and Empowerment (S.C.A.R.E.) have links nationwide. These groups are working to raise awareness of the needs of the sickle cell patient while reaching out to patients and families.

THE AMERICAN SICKLE CELL ANEMIA ASSOCIATION

This organization provides a wide range of services to people with either sickle cell trait or variants of the disease itself—and to their families. Key services include: ongoing follow-up diagnostic testing, counseling, and tracking services for parents with infants who screen positive, family counseling and support services, coordination of medical, social services, education and support for the program's clientele, teacher education and screening services at upwards of seventy-five local health fairs. In addition, ASCAA has outreach programs to the region's African American, Hispanic, Mediterranean, and Arab communities for family education and the identification of incidence of sickle cell disease.

American Sickle Cell Anemia Association
PO Box 1971
10300 Carnegie Avenue
Cleveland, Ohio 44106
Phone: (216) 229-8600 Contact: Ira Bragg
Fax: (216) 229-4500
URL: http://www.ascaa.org
e-mail:ashc@cybernex.net

THE SICKLE CELL DISEASE ASSOCIATION OF AMERICA

The goal of the Sickle Cell Disease Association of America (SCDAA) is "to find a cure and improve the quality of life for those who are afflicted and their families." The SCDAA publishes and distributes to parents and teachers educational materials for living and coping with sickle cell disease.

Through its member organizations, SCDAA provides such services as screening and referrals, counseling, home nursing care, research updates, psycho-social services, transportation, summer camp, local and regional workshops, international symposiums, as well as a sickle cell chat room. The SCDAA also provides guidelines for starting local sickle cell groups.

Sickle Cell Disease Association of America
200 Corporate Pointe, Suite 495
Culver City, California 90230-8727
Office (310) 216-6363
Fax (310) 215-3722
General Public (800) 421-8453
e-mail: scdaa@sicklecelldisease.org
website: www.sicklecelldisease.org

SICKLE CELL ADVOCATES FOR RESEARCH AND EMPOWERMENT

Sickle Cell Advocates for Research and Empowerment, Inc. (S.C.A.R.E.) is built around the concept of the sickle cell "defier." The defier is an active, responsible participant in his or her own care, and is also an advocate for the sickle cell community.

S.C.A.R.E. reaches out to sickle cell patients, their family, friends. and health care providers, stressing the importance of education and personal involvement in fighting sickle cell disease.

On their "always under construction" website, S.C.A.R.E., like its sister organizations, provides links to sickle cell organizations around the world. These links are in categories like:

- links to medical information
- empowerment support
- alternative healing options
- research updates
- activist updates
- coping resources
- a sickle cell community rolodex

S.C.A.R.E. also offers a sickle cell bulletin board ("Coollist") where meetings, events, and announcements of interest to the sickle cell community are posted. You'll find it at http://coollist.com.

At "Coollist" you'll also find people talking together about such topics as diet, exercise, and alternative medicine.

Sickle Cell Advocates for Research and Empowerment, Inc.
  (S.C.A. R. E.)
Ivor Balin Pannell , President
Deborah G. Oster Pannell, Secy, Treas.
PO Box 630127
Bronx, New York 10463
Phone/Fax (718) 884-9670
SCAREemail@defiers.com
website: http://www.defiers.com

OTHER RESOURCES

There are many other organizations, foundations and groups that offer support to the sickle cell patient. A brief list follows:

The Sickle Cell Information Center
P.O. Box 109, Grady Memorial Hospital

80 Butler Street SE
Atlanta, GA 30303
Phone: 404-616-3572
Fax: 404-66-5998
e-mail: aplatt@emory.edu
website: http://www.emory.edu/PEDS/SICKLE;
    www.SCINFO.org; www.sickleCellKids.org

The Sickle Cell Foundation of Georgia, Inc.
2391 Benjamin E. Mays Dr. SW
Atlanta, GA 30311
Phone: 404-755-1641
Fax: 404-755-7955
e-mail: sicklefg@mindspring.com
website: www.mindspring.com/-sicklefg
D. Jean Brannan, President/CEO

The African American Community Health Network (AACHN)
The Emerald City Seventh Day Adventist Church
The Holgate Church of Christ
2600 South Holgate
801-25th Street
Seattle, Washington

The Keon Paschal Perry Sickle Cell Anemia Disease
    Awareness, Inc.
(KPPSCADA) Contact:
Sickle Cell Anemia Disease Awareness, Inc.
Perry Building
7510 Granby Street, Suite 207
Norfolk, Virginia 23505

The Sickle Cell Anemia Research Foundation
2625 3rd Street
Alexandria, Louisiana 71302

Fax (318) 487-9990
e-mail: rgmscarf@aol.com

The Wellness Web Parent's Sickle Cell Information page at
http://wellweb.com/INDEX/QSICKLE.HTM

The National Center for Education in Maternal and Child
   Health
2000 15th Street N, Suite 701
Arlington, Virginia 22201-2617
(703) 524-7802

The National Association for Sickle Cell Disease, Inc.
3345 Wilshire Blvd.
Los Angeles, California 90010-1880
Phone: (800) 421-8453 Contact: Pamela
Fax: (213) 736-5211

The Alliance of Genetic Support Groups
4301 Connecticut Avenue NW, Suite 404
Washington, DC 20008-2304
(202) 966-5557
(800) 336-4363
e-mail: info@geneticalliance.org
Website: geneticalliance.org/

Local March of Dimes Chapters (listed in your phone directory)

National Heart, Lung, and Blood Institute (NHLB), a part of the
   Federal Government's National Institutes of Health, at
   http://www.nhlbi.nih.gov/

Sickle Cell Disease Scientific Research Group
6701 Rockledge Drive, MSC 7950
Bethesda, MD 20892-7950

301-435-0055 (voice)
301-480-0868 (fax).

NIH Sickle Cell Center's website at
   http://www.rhofed.com/sickle.
This site lists all of the federally funded centers with e-mail
   addresses and locations.

Sickle Cell Disease Association of America
200 Corporate Point #945,
Culver City, CA 90230-7633
1- 800-421-8453, 310-216-6363
FAX 310-215-3722.
A state by state listing of member chapters where you can obtain
   sickle cell information and local referrals is located on their
   website at: http://www.sicklecelldisease.org/programs.htm

Genetic Disease Resource Center
California State Department of Health Services
2151 Berkeley Way, Annex 4
Berkeley, CA 94704
510-540-2534

STOP STUDY—Stroke Prevention Centers at
   http://www.neuro.mcg.edu/cvhp/STOP/centers.html. These
   centers can perform Transcranial Doppler ultrasound to detect
   those children at high risk of having a stroke.

Council of Regional Networks for Genetic Services—CORN.
   This is a great resource for genetics in the US including sickle
   cell clinics, testing locations and conferences. At
   http://www.cc.emory.edu/PEDIATRICS/corn/member/regions.
   htm

The Georgia Comprehensive Sickle Cell Center at Grady Health
System in Atlanta. The world's first 24-hour acute care clinic
dedicated to patients with sickle syndromes. Health maintenance clinics for children and adults.
James R. Eckman, M.D.,
Director The Sickle Cell Information Center
http://www.emory.edu/PEDS/SICKLE; www/SCINO.org;
www.SickleCellKids.org
80 Butler Street, S.E. P.O. Box 109
Atlanta, GA 30335
phone 404-616-3572 Fax 404-616-5998

SICKLE CELL WEB RESOURCES

The Sickle Cell Information Center at
http://www.emory.edu/PEDS/SICKLE

This is a comprehensive sickle cell site based at The Georgia
Comprehensive Sickle Cell Center at Grady Health System in
Atlanta, Georgia. In 1984, Grady Memorial Hospital opened the
world's first twenty-four-hour comprehensive acute care Sickle
Cell Center. The goals of the Center were to provide twenty-four-
hour acute care in a designated area with a dedicated staff, provide
health care consultation, research new treatments, and provide
education, and support services to residents of the state of Georgia
with sickle cell syndromes. The mission of the web site is to provide
sickle cell patient and professional education, news, research
updates and world wide sickle cell resources. Email consultations
are now provided to patients and clinicians in countries around the
world. All email questions are reviewed by a physician assistant and
answered or sent to the appropriate medical staff for a reply.

Current content areas include: sickle cell overview for the lay
audience, an overview for providers, research updates, a list of
sickle cell clinics and centers, web links, a download PowerPoint
tutorial, a frequently asked questions page, and a means of submit-

ting email questions. The web site contains sections for health care providers including two online clinical management books, research updates, conference information web links, and news. The sections for patients and family members contain articles in lay terms, a frequently asked questions page, down load educational coloring books, and locations of sickle cell clinics nationwide. There is an extensive list of links to other sickle cell websites. There is a resource page with recommended books, videos, monographs and CD-ROMs. Worldwide sickle cell educational conferences are posted. There is an informational guide for teachers and employers to help sickle cell patients with basic pain prevention measures.

The Globin Gene Server
http://globin.cse.psu.edu/
This site provides data and tools for studying the function of DNA sequences, with an emphasis on those involved in the production of hemoglobin. There is an online copy of *A Syllabus of Human Hemoglobin Variants* (1996) and most of *A Syllabus of Thalassemia Mutations* (1997) .

The CDC Sickle Cell Statistical Page
http://www.cdc.gov/genetics/hugenet/reviews/sickle.htm
This site has sickle cell statistical information with incidence and prevalence of complications.

University of Rochester Medical Center Hemoglobinopathies Brochures and Fact Sheets
http://www.urmc.rochester.edu/smd/genetics/hemobroc.htm
This site has fact sheets on hemoglobinopathies.

Sickle Cell Disease in Newborns and Infants
http://wellweb.com/INDEX/QSICKLE.HTM
A Guide for Parents—National Library of Medicine for lay audiences. An excellent guide.

Sickle Cell Disease Association of America (SCDAA)
http://www.sicklecelldisease.org/

This is the home page for the Sickle Cell Disease Association of America, Inc., representing the many community sickle cell organizations across the nation. There is a list of educational materials for purchase, locations of member organizations, and sickle cell news.

Sickle Cell Kids
http://www.SickleCellKids.org

This is a kid friendly site full of sickle cell information in a fun, animated site. There are games, stories, letters from celebrities and more. The staff of the Sickle Cell Center in Atlanta provide the scientific content.

Harvard School of Medicine Joint Center for Sickle Cell and Thalassemia
http://sickle.bwh.harvard.edu

This excellent site has information for clinicians and patients. There are very good articles about current issues in sickle cell treatment and links to other sickle cell sites.

The Comprehensive Sickle Cell Centers—Statistical Coordination Web Site http://www.rhofed.com/sickle/

This site has information on the ten NIH funded comprehensive sickle cell centers. There are links to other sickle cell sites and information about ongoing research in the ten centers.

Washington University Biology Department Sickle Cell Web Page
http://www.nslc.wustl.edu/courses/Bio296A/allen/sicklecell/
sicklecell.html.

This is an excellent site for students and patients. A case study, Discovery and Biological Basis, Molecular Biology of Sickle Celled Hemoglobin, Biogeography and Ecology of Sickle Celled Anemia, Treatment and Political Aspects are all sections for review. The graphics and questions are excellent.

Sickle Cell Kids
http://www.SicklecellKids.org
This demonstration version of the new web site for sickle cell education and inspiration is up for viewing.

Sickle Cell Advocates for Research and Empowerment (S.C.A.R.E.)
http://www.defiers.com/
In 1997 Deborah and Ivor Pannell formed Sickle Cell Advocates for Research and Empowerment (S. C. A. R. E.) whose primary aim is to equip the sickle cell community with up-to-date information that encourages advocacy and self-empowerment. The site includes everything from "Research News" to the personal experiences of "BloodSongs," as well as a comprehensive listing of links.

The American Pain Society
http://www.ampainsoc.org/
This organization has published "Sickle Cell Pain Guideline" and has many pain management resources.

The National Library of Medicine Medline
http://www.nlm.nih.gov/
Free Medline searching of the latest publications in the medical press.

CD ROMS

The Wellcome Trust Presents: Topics in International Health—Sickle Cell Disease. The health series on Sickle Cell Disease is a comprehensive review for health care professionals, students, researchers and teachers. For information and ordering see http://www.cabi.org or http://www.wellcome.ac.uk

The Sickle Cell Information Center CD ROM
http://www.emory.edu/PEDS/SICKLE
This CD has a copy of the internet web site, an online copy of this book, and PowerPoint slide shows for use in teaching and printing. There is a database template for storing patient information in Microsoft Access.

Sickle Cell Rap Music—Teaching CD—A wonderful teaching tool produced by two family practice physicians, the Clarke brothers, for children and teens. The CDs and further information are available from the Clarke brothers on the Internet at www.mdmdinc.com, by e-mail at StopAsthma@AOL.com or by phone at (917) 208-2467.

StarBright Sickle Cell—Discovery Series CD ROM—This excellent resource for children and teens teaches preventive health habits, all about common blood tests, IVs, and x rays. This is available for free to patients and families upon request from Starbright at http://www.starbright.com

BOOKS

Understanding Sickle Cell Disease by **Miriam Bloom, Ph.D.** This is an excellent book written for lay audiences by the former senior editor for the *Journal of the National Cancer Institute*. The book is well organized and contains current information explaining the origins, complications, treatments and the future of research for sickle cell disease. It is excellent for patients, parents, and lay audiences interested in sickle cell. The book is available from University Press Books, 601-982-1800, and online at http://www.sci-write.com/sickle.html

The New England Regional Genetics Group (NERGG) Monographs on Sickle Cell Related Pain Assessment and Management. These guidebooks were the results of a conference in 1993. These booklets detail pain assessment methods, sickle cell pain treatment and prevention strategies:
1) *Sickle Cell Related Pain : Assessment and Management, A Guide for Patients and Parents.*
2) *Quick Clinical Reference Guide for Health Care Providers*
3) *Sickle Cell Related Pain: Assessment and Management, Conference Proceedings.*
Contact NERGG at 207-288-2704 or their website at http://www.acadia.net/nergg/booklets.html

A Parents Handbook for Sickle Cell Disease Part 1, Birth to Six Years of Age, Part 2, Six to Eighteen Years of Age. Shellye Lessing, MS and Elliott Vinchinsky, M.D., eds. Children's Hospital — Oakland Sickle Cell Center. Available at the Maternal Child Clearing House phone 1-888-434-4624. This is an excellent handbook for parents.

N.I.H. Management of Sicle Cell Disease. Available as download at http://www.nhlbi.nih.gov/health/pros/blood/sickle/index.htm. An excellent updated guidebook for health care providers from the nation's top experts.

Sickle Cell Disease: Comprehensive Screening and Management in Newborns and Infants (AHCPR Guidelines 93-0562, and 93-0563). This is a 1993 guidebook for health care providers that details early child care and newborn screening for sickle cell. Phone 1-800-358-9295.

Acute Pain Management in Infants, Children and Adolescents. Operative and Medical Procedures (AHCPR Guidelines 92-0020, 92-0032, 92-0019). Phone 1-800-358-9295. A guide to help clinicians assess and manage pain.

Medical Guide for Heath Care Providers—Management and Therapy of Sickle Cell Disease, N.I.H. Publication 95-2117, Third edition 1995. Clarice Reid M.D. et al., eds. A guidebook written for health care providers by the leading experts in sickle cell disease to help manage the most common problems in sickle cell patients. Published in 1995, a new update is in the works. This can be viewed online at the Sickle Cell Information Center website.

About Sickle Cell Disease and Sickle Cell Trait. Channing L Bete Inc. Publication number 38992A-12-94. Phone 1-800-628-7733. This is a public-patient informational brochure with fifteen pages of text and illustrations for the lay audience. Spanish version publication number 39339A-8-95 is also available.

Sickle Cell Disease—Basic Principles and Clinical Practice. Stephen Embury et al., eds. Raven Press 1994. ISBN 0-7817-0142-2, order code 2764. A comprehensive medical textbook for health care providers by many of the world's leading sickle cell experts.

Sickle Cell Disease, Third Edition. Graham Serjeant, M.D. Oxford Press 2001. ISBN 0-19-263036-9. This is one of the most comprehensive medical textbooks in the world. Dr. Serjeant spent much of his medical career caring for sickle cell patients in Jamaica and has traveled around the world as a sickle cell consultant. This text is written for medical personnel, but it is the one reference book to have on the shelf. www.oup.co.uk

Puzzles by Dava Walker
Puzzles is a story about Cassie, a school-age child with sickle cell disease. This book for children is available from Carolina Wren Press at (919) 560-2738. ISBN 0-914996-29-0. There is a 30% discount for schools, hospitals, clinics, libraries, and other non-profit agencies.

My Life with Sickle Cell Disease by Walter Elwood Brandon
Walter Elwood Brandon, the co-founder of the Sickle Cell Genetic
Disease Council ISEPA, now known as The Sickle Cell Disease
Association of America/ Philadelphia-Delaware Valley, has survived
the trauma of living with Sickle Cell Disease for over half a century. For additional information or orders call (215) 471-8686 or fax
order to (215) 471-7441. Address: Sickle Cell Disease Association
of America Philadelphia/ Delaware Valley Chapter, 4601 Market
Street, Philadelphia, PA 19139.

Transfusion Support in Patients with Sickle Cell Disease. From the
American Association of Blood Banks. The authors of this clinically
focused book review the current knowledge and practices in transfusing patients with sickle cell disease to assist clinicians in understanding the complex role transfusion plays in treatment of this disease. 1998; 398 pp, hardbound, ISBN 0-931092-22-1. Order Form
at http://www.halcyon.com/iasp/sickle.html

Sickle Cell Pain Progress in Pain Research and Management, v.11, by
Samir K. Ballas. 1998; 398 pp, hardbound, ISBN 0-931092-22-1.
Order Form at http://www.halcyon.com/iasp/sickle.html

**Guideline for the Management of Acute and Chronic Pain in Sickle
Cell Disease (From American Pain Society).** 1999. This is an excellent handbook focusing on pain assessment and treatment. The
review is evidence based and peer reviewed by many experts in
sickle cell disease. Contact: American Pain Society, 4700 W. Lake
Avenue, Glenview, IL 60025. Tel 847/375-4715; Fax 847-375-6315;
e-mail info@ampainsoc.org Web site: http://www.ampainsoc.org/

A Guide to Sickle Cell Disease—an 86-page paperback reference
with color pictures and guides for common problems. The Sickle
Cell Trust and Dr. Graham Serjeant in Jamaica. $30. Address: 14
Milverton Crescent, Kingston 6, Jamaica, West Indies. Phone 876-
970-0077 Fax 876-970-0074 e-mail grserjeant@cwjamaica.com

Sickle Cell Disease. Susan Dudley Gold. A 48-page book for families and older children. The feature of the book is Keon Penn, the first sickle cell patient to undergo unrelated cord blood stem cell transplant. Enslow Publishers, 2001, $18.95.

Sickle Cell Anemia. Alvin and Virginia Silverstein and Laura Silverstein Nunn. A 112-page book for families and patients. It is easy to read and understand. Enslow Publishers, 1997, $20.95

Dying in the City of Blues, Sickle Cell Anemia and the Politics of Race and Health. Keith Wailoo. This is a 360 page description of the history, social, cultural, and political aspects of sickle cell disease in Memphis, TN. University of North Carolina Press, 2001, $16.95 paperback, $34.95 hardback.

VIDEOS—SLIDES

Sickle Cell Disease. An overview for parents and children. Distributed by Medical Audio Visual Communications, this excellent twenty-minute video gives the basics about the disease, complications and preventive treatment. Call 1-800-757-4868.

Sickle Cell Provider Course. A ten-hour video for health care providers. This CME accredited video course is sponsored by Emory University and the Georgia Comprehensive Sickle Cell Center. For more information, visit the Sickle Cell Information Web Site at http://www.emory.edu/PEDS/SICKLE

Sickle Cell Pain Management Video Course. A five-hour CME accredited video course sponsored by Emory University and the Georgia Comprehensive Sickle Cell Center For more information, visit the Sickle Cell Information Website at http://www.emory.edu/PEDS/SICKLE

Living with Sickle Cell Disease. A twenty-seven-minute VHS video produced by the Sickle Cell Trust and Dr. Graham Serjeant in Jamaica. $30. Address: 14 Milverton Crescent, Kingston 6, Jamaica, West Indies. Phone 876-970-0077 Fax 876-970-0074 email grserjeant@cwjamaica.com

Sickle Cell Teaching Slide Sets. There are thirty-five 35mm slides in each of two sets: 1. Clinical Features demonstrating common complications. 2. Epidemiology—Sickle cell around the world. $100 each or $185 for both sets. The Sickle Cell Trust and Dr. Graham Serjeant in Jamaica. Address: 14 Milverton Crescent, Kingston 6, Jamaica, West Indies. Phone 876-970-0077 Fax 876-970-0074, e-mail grserjeant@cwjamaica.com

MEETINGS

There are two annual national meetings: The N.I.H. Sickle Cell Center's meeting in the spring and the Sickle Cell Disease Association's meeting in the fall. Visit the Conference information page on the Sickle Cell Information Web Site at http://www.emory.edu/PEDS/SICKLE

CLINICS

The national and international list of clinics with sickle cell services is growing daily. Please check the latest list on the Sickle Cell Informational web site at www.emory.edu/PEDS/SICKLE/ Clinics.htm. If you cannot find a clinic near you , ask other patients and supporters about where they obtain good medical care. If you have no patients or sickle cell associations to ask, start with the nearest hematologist, followed by your pediatrician. It is worthwhile to establish annual contact with a large sickle cell center to keep informed about the latest advances and have an established relationship if you have a complicated problem.

HEALTH PASSPORT
MEDICAL INFORMATION TO KEEP

Name:_____

Date of Birth:_____

Sickle Cell Type (SS,SC, SBth):_____

Medical Record Number:_____

Allergies:_____

Medications:_____

Physician:_____

Phone:_____

Complications:_____

_____

_____

Transfusions:_____

Surgeries:_____

Pain Medications:_____

ER Pain Medications_____

DICTIONARY

Acute Chest Syndrome—When sickle red blood cells block blood flow to the lungs. This can cause chest pain, shortness of breath and cough. It is treated in the hospital with blood transfusions.

Amniocentesis—A test done by taking a small amount of fluid from the womb of a pregnant woman to determine if the baby has sickle cell disease or another genetic problem.

Anemia—a low red blood cell count. Anemia can be caused by many different events including sickle cell disease.

Aplastic Anemia—Decreased red blood cell count due to the bone marrow factory shutting down. The most common cause is a virus called Parvo B19.

Bone Marrow—The blood factory inside of your big bones that makes red blood cells, white blood cells and platelets.

Bone Marrow Transplant—A procedure that kills the existing bone marrow factory and plants donor (usually a matched brother or sister) marrow by transfusion. The bone begins to make blood cells according to the genetic code of the donor. This has cured several sickle cell patients.

Carrier—One who inherits only one gene for a genetic problem like sickle cell. Usually there are no symptoms, and the carrier will never have the disease. Two carriers have a 25 percent risk of having a child with disease.

Chromosome—The DNA code for all the parts of the human body. Each person has forty-six individual chromosomes in cells, twenty-three donated from each parent. Chromosome 11 is where the sickle cell mutation occurs.

CBC—Complete Blood Count—a blood test that gives clinicians information about how many red cells, white cells, and platelets a person has in her bloodstream.

Folic Acid—Folate—a B vitamin necessary for making new red blood cells. Most sickle cell patients should take 1mg a day. It is found in green leafy vegetables, cereals.

Gall Bladder—a pouch in the right upper abdomen under the liver. It stores bile to help digest fats in the diet.

Gall Stones—Too much bilirubin from red blood cell breakdown can cause stones to form in the gall bladder. This can cause pain in the right upper abdomen, nausea and indigestion when eating fatty foods. The gall bladder can be removed if it is full of stones.

Genes—These are the basic units of inheritance. They are located on chromosomes.

Gene Therapy—Treatment that will change the genetic defect in sickle cell disease. This is experimental at this time.

Hand—Foot Syndrome or Dactylitis—Swelling and pain in the hands and feet usually seen in six month to three-year old sickle cell patients.

Hemoglobin—The protein substance inside the red blood cells that holds and releases oxygen. This is where the sickle mutation occurs.

Hemoglobin Electrophoresis—The blood test that identifies the type of hemoglobins present in the red blood cells.

Hemoglobin AS—this is sickle cell trait. The inheritance of a normal A hemoglobin gene and a sickle hemoglobin gene.

Hemoglobin S Beta Thalassemia—This is a type of sickle cell disease where one inherits a S gene and a beta thalassemia gene from each parent. S beta zero thalassemia is more severe than s beta plus thalassemia.

Hemoglobin SC—A type of sickle cell disease in which one inherits a S gene and a C gene from each parent. This causes sickle cell complications with increased eye and bone problems. Life expectancy is longer than with hemoglobin SS.

Hemoglobin SS—This is called sickle cell anemia and is the most common form of sickle cell disease.

Hemolysis—the breaking apart of red blood cells. Normal red cells last 120 days, sickle red blood cells last about fourteen days.

Hydroxyurea—hydrea, for short, is the first medication that increases fetal hemoglobin. It reduces by one half pain events, the need for hospital admissions, and the need for blood transfusions.

IV—Intravenous—a small plastic catheter placed in a vein to allow water, blood, or medication to enter the blood stream directly.

Jaundice—a yellow color in the white part (sclera) of the eye produced by increased bilirubin in the blood. Usually caused by increased red blood cell breakdown in sickle cell patients.

MRI—Magnetic Resonance Imaging—a large magnet based device that painlessly creates images of the brain and other organs of the body

Pain Episode or "Crisis"—Pain in the bones and muscles where blood flow has been blocked by sickled red blood cells.

Portacath—an under-the-skin port that allows one time needle sticks and venous access to draw blood samples and give fluids, blood, and medications.

Spleen—An organ in the left upper area of the stomach that helps filter germs from the blood stream.

Sequestration—Blocked blood flow from sickled red blood cells in the spleen or liver. Blood can flow in but it cannot flow out. This causes abdominal pain, swelling and weakness.

Stroke—Blocked blood flow to an area of the brain that can cause weakness, numbness, trouble speaking, or trouble thinking.

Transcranial Doppler—TCD—a special ultrasound device that uses painless sound waves to check for blocked blood flow in the brain. This test can identify children at greatest risk of having a stroke.

SCHOLARSHIPS

The Sickle Cell Disease Association of America
200 Corporate Point #945
Culver City, CA 90230-7633
Phone 1- 800-421-8453 , 310-216-6363
FAX 310-215-3722

A state by state listing of member chapters where you can obtain local chapter scholarship information located on their website at: http://www.sicklecelldisease.org

The International Association of Sickle Cell Nurses and Physician Assistants (IASCNAPA) IASCNAPA
c/o Deborah Boger
Wake Forrest University—Baptist Medical Center
Department of Pediatrics
Medical Center Blvd
Winston-Salem, NC 27157-1081

APPENDIX I

The History of Sickle Cell Disease and Distribution

HEMOGLOBINOPATHIES

A mutation or change in the DNA code blueprint can cause genetic diseases.

Hemoglobinopathies are a group of genetic diseases that occur because of a mutation in the DNA blueprint that directs the making of hemoglobin. The importance of hemoglobin is that it is the main carrier of oxygen in the body. Only 1 percent of the wide variety of hemoglobinopathies can cause serious diseases such as sickle cell disease and the thalassemias. Thus, you and I can carry a hemoglobin gene abnormality and not know about it because it does not show itself as disease.

SCIENTISTS LEARN HOW WE INHERIT GENETIC DEFECTS

Sometimes we take knowledge for granted, without honoring the human effort that went into gaining it. Let's correct that by going back in time, to see how we learned that hemoglobinopathies are inherited from our parents.

HEMOPHILIA

The story begins in the 19th century, when a simple but very damaging blood disorder called *hemophilia* plagued royal families, though only the males were afflicted by it. Hemophilia leads to massive bleeding when an injury occurs inside or outside the body. Without treatment, the hemophiliac can die of bleeding from even minor wounds.

Treatment for hemophilia means transfusion, but blood transfusion wasn't available at this time. And without the benefits of transfusion, most hemophiliacs, even royal ones, easily bled to death.

GREGOR MENDEL AND THE BIRTH OF GENETICS

In 1865, an Austrian monk named Gregor Mendel proposed that discrete units he called *factors* (later to be called *genes)* are passed down among family members to produce particular observable characteristics he called traits.

The scientific community didn't immediately act on Mendel's theory. Part of the problem was the novelty of the ideas. First, Mendel had presented his now famous garden pea experiments in a mathematical model. The math was simple enough, but biologists at that time were not used to interpreting experiments in mathematical terms.

There was a second reason for the gap between Mendel's work and the important work that followed from it. The very concept of cell division, crucial to Mendel's theory, had not yet been discovered. In fact, it was still unknown when Mendel died in 1884.

GENETIC BASIS OF HEMOGLOBINOPATHIES— THE HISTORY OF SICKLE CELL

The story of discovering hemoglobinopathies is exciting. It shows how one observant mind can change our understanding of an entire field of study.

Sickle cell disease has probably been in the world for thousands of years. There are African writings that described the symptoms of sickle cell and gave it names like *chwecheechwe, abututuo, nuidudui* and *nwiiwii*. The first published reports of sickle cell disease in African medical literature were in the 1870s. The first American case described was that of Walter Clement Noel, a first-year dental student at the Chicago College of Dental Surgery. Noel was admitted to the Presbyterian Hospital in late 1904. Ernest E. Irons, a 27-year-old intern, obtained Noel's history and performed routine physical, blood, and urine examinations. Irons noticed that Noel's blood smear contained "many pear-shaped and elongated forms" and alerted his attending physician, James B. Herrick, to the unusual blood findings. Irons drew a rough sketch of these erythrocytes in the hospital record. Herrick and Irons followed Noel over the next two-and-a-half years through several episodes of severe illness. Then, Noel returned to Grenada to practice dentistry. He died nine years later at the age of thirty-two.

Seven years after Herrick's and Iron's discovery, V.E. Emmel reported in the *Archives of Internal Medicine* that the sickling observed by James Herrick occurred both in healthy individuals (with sickle trait) and in people who had anemia (sickle cell disease).

Later, two researchers, Gillespie and Haln, demonstrated that it was a reduction in the oxygen content of the blood that led to the sickling of the red blood cells observed by James Herrick. It was Haln who first used the phrase "sickle cell trait" to describe those healthy individuals who had some sickling of red blood cells but no apparent anemia.

By the 1940s, sickle cell disease had already become the most thoroughly studied genetic disease in medical literature. Linus Pauling demonstrated, by comparing normal and sickle hemoglobin, that abnormal hemoglobin was the cause of sickle cell disease.

The big question remained: "What was the abnormality in sickle hemoglobin?" Pauling knew there was an abnormality in the hemoglobin chain, but where in the chain did the abnormality occur and what was its exact nature?

The answer to this question came in the 1950s from an American scientist named Vernon Ingram. It was already known that hemoglobin, like any other protein, is made up of small units bound together into amino acids. The twenty types of amino acids can arrange themselves in different sequences to form all sorts of proteins. Some proteins become bone, others become skin, etc.

What Dr. Ingram did was painstakingly to arrange—without benefit of the automated gene sequencers we have today—in their exact order the amino acids that make up hemoglobin. In this way Ingram showed for the first time that an amino acid called *valine* had replaced another amino acid called *glutamic* in the sixth position of the beta globin chain of hemoglobin. This very small change, as we all know now, had very great impact on the lives of people who suffer from it.

DNA AND THE GENETIC CODE

We've told you something about genetics by telling you part of the history that made the science of genetics possible. Now it's time to talk about the genetic code itself.

In the famous "fly room" at Columbia University in New York City, Thomas Morgan, in 1910, while working on the now familiar fruit fly, discovered that genes are carried in chromosomes. Only in 1944 did researchers at Rockefeller Institute in New York find out precisely what genes are when they discovered them to be made of deoxyribonucleic acid (DNA).

In 1953, two young men, James Watson and Francis Crick. working at Cambridge University in England, carried this work a significant step further by uncovering the nature of the DNA molecule itself. The DNA, they noted, contains sugars, phosphates and bases which are arranged in a spiral, complementary fashion, which they termed the "double helix." The DNA itself, in the nucleus of the molecule, provides a blueprint for the making of protein in the cytoplasm.

The work of Watson and Crick was one of the great scientific discoveries of all time—a discovery that scientists knew at once could change our species by giving us the ability to deliberately alter our own genes. But like all big answers, Watson's and Crick's discoveries led to a new big question: How is information carried from the DNA in the nucleus into the cytoplasm to make the proteins?

The answer came in 1960 when Sydney Brenner, Matthew Meselson, and Francois Jacob learned that the information is carried through another acid called RNA (ribonucleic acid). RNA is coded by the DNA in a process called *transcription*. It is then taken into the cytoplasm from the nucleus. Here RNA becomes an insider that carries exactly the same configuration as the DNA. The RNA becomes the template on which proteins are designed, in a process called *translation*, according to "specs" laid out by the DNA. For that reason RNA is sometimes called *messenger RNA*.

One of the breath-taking facts about this process of coding and uncoding is that it uses only four letters. Just as all the information contained in this book is written in just twenty-six letters of the alphabet and so is all of the *Encyclopedia Britannica*, and the works of Mark Twain and Langston Hughes, so in life sciences, all creatures are formed from just four letters. No matter the size of the creature, be it as small as the hepatitis virus or as big and eloquent as Martin Luther King Jr., it is formed from just four letters. These four letters, known as A,C, T, and G, are the code for all the twenty amino acids that form the hundreds of thousands of different proteins that make up the whole body.

In the human DNA structure, A,C,T,G are arranged in a helix several billion units in length. This means that there is great opportunity for error. While the vast majority of human beings are born normal, an impressive number of pregnancies do end up in miscarriage. This is because fetuses that have severe genetic diseases, incompatible with life, abort naturally within the first three months of pregnancy. If the genetic disease is mild or moderate and compatible with life, the fetus has a good chance of being born and surviving. Sickle cell disease falls into this latter category.

NATURE OF MUTATIONS

A misarrangement of DNA bases may involve only one letter out of the more than 3 billion, a misarrangement as simple as the absence of the correct letter in its proper position (scientists call this deletion) or insertion of an incorrect base in a wrong position (scientist call this substitution). Such a simple mistake leads to placing an amino acid in the wrong position in the sequence of a protein, and can alter the physical characteristics of that protein so that it is incapable of carrying out its function.

In sickle hemoglobin there is incorrect placement of the amino acid valine instead of glutamic acid in the 6th position of the hemoglobin protein. One "mistake" changes the physical characteristics of the hemoglobin molecule in such a way that when oxygen tension is low (such as during exercise) the hemoglobin becomes insoluble instead of soluble. The insoluble hemoglobin makes the red blood cells sickle and become stiff instead of being soft and pliable. As a result, they block the vessels, starving many tissues of oxygen.

An underlying theme of all this is that genes determine the formation of our proteins, and proteins are highly organized structures that essentially determine who we are. Proteins determine every aspect of human endeavor—abilities, drive, behavior, appearance, how we react to the external environment, and how we age.

We all know or have read about human beings who achieve tremendous feats in sports, business, academics, or someone who had a spontaneous remission from a serious disease such as cancer or AIDS. Such extraordinary things occur because one person makes proteins which other people cannot make.

Except for identical twins, no two individuals are alike. Each is unique. That's another feature of this dazzling system: each new human body modifies the genes it inherits so as to make different proteins. It is the capacity to make different proteins that gives us our human individuality.

We said earlier that big new answers make for big new questions. The question scientists are working to answer today, in a work that is known as the Human Genome Project, is how many proteins there are and what the function of each of them is. A rough map of this universal guide to the genetic make-up of human beings has already been drawn, but it will take many decades before all the details are filled in. The impact of this project on our understanding of ourselves and on our ability to shape our human destinies remains beyond our imagination.

GENETICS OF HEMOGLOBIN

From the viewpoint of an individual affected by them, some departures from "normal" genetic coding seem like errors, because they produce genetic "defects." These, in turn, may produce human beings in some sense "disabled." But from a wider viewpoint, such departures—we call them *mutations*—aren't mistakes at all. They're creative experiments. Some changes may worsen or have no effect on our chances for survival as a species. Others may produce the brilliant originality necessary to create some important work of art or make a scientific discovery.

We believe that the sickle cell mutation, where it first occurred in West Africa, allowed human beings who lived there, and therefore their gene pool, to better survive the threat of malaria. The most effective form of the mutation is sickle cell trait (hemoglobin S mutation) in which less than 50 percent of the body's hemoglobin has this arrangement. Those with sickle cell trait still get malaria, a red blood cell parasite, but they survive malaria better than those without the trait.

Unfortunately for us, the existence of the trait made the disease possible. By mating, two people with sickle cell trait may produce offspring with sickle cell disease.

SICKLE HEMOGLOBIN
INCIDENCE

In the Black population in the United States, the incidence of hemoglobin S trait or sickle cell trait is approximately 8 percent or about one in twelve individuals. The incidence of hemoglobin C trait is about 3 percent, and of beta thalassemia trait, almost 1.5 percent. The estimates of the incidence of sickle cell syndromes is: sickle cell anemia (Hb SS), 1 in every 375 live Black births; sickle cell hemoglobin C disease (Hb SC), 1 in every 833 Black births; and sickle cell beta thalassemia (Hb S beta thal), 1 in every 1667 Black births.

THE DISTRIBUTION

Sickle cell syndromes occur in higher frequency in people from geographic areas where malaria was endemic. This occurs because carriers, like those with sickle cell trait, appear to have some protection against severe malaria infection. These genes are found most often in Africans, Arabs, Egyptians, Turks, Greeks, Italians, Iranians, and Asiatic Indians. In the United States, which the disease is more common in African Americans, while it is seen in individuals of almost every ethnic background.

WORLD WIDE VIEW

Sickle cell disease is found in many countries around the world as populations have moved from place to place. Africa still has the highest incidence of trait and disease with the incidence of sickle cell trait approaching 60 percent in some areas around the equator. Other territories around the world and the incidence of sickle trait are:

India—9%-38%
Southern Italy—10%
Greece—8%-27%
Brazil—7%-10%
Venezuela—11%
Cuba—5%
Puerto Rico—5%
Panama—12%-14%
Saudi Arabia—5%-25%
Surinam—15%
Jamaica—10%
West Africa—15%-25%
Curacao—12%

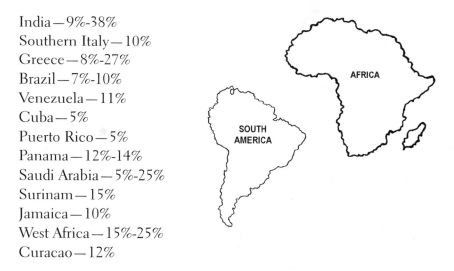

APPENDIX II

Bibliography

Adeodu OO, Alimi T, Adekile AD. A comprehensive study of the perception of sickle cell anemia by married Nigerian rural and urban women. Complications of sickle cell trait. *West Afr J Med* 2000 Jan-Mar; *19*(1):1–5.

Aldrich TK, Dhuper SK, Patwa WS, Makolo E, Suzuka SM, Najeebi SA, Santhanakrishnan S, Nagel RL, Fabry ME. Pulmonary entrapment of sickle cells: the role of regional alveolar hypoxia. *J Appl Physiol* 1996; *80*(2):531–539.

Alegre M-L, Gastadello K, Abramovicz D, Kinnaert P, Vereerstraeten P, DePauw L, Vandenabeele P, Moser M, Leo O, Goldman M. Evidence that pentoxifylline reduces anti-CD3 monoclonal antibody-induced cytokine release syndrome. *Transplantation* 1991; *52*(4):674–679.

Al-Salem AH, Oaisruddin S. The significance of biliary sludge in children with sickle cell disease. *Pediatr Surg Int* 1998 Jan; *13*(1):14–16.

Aluoch JR. Higher resistance to Plasmodium falciparum infection in patients with homozygous sickle cell disease in western Kenya. *Trop Med Int Health* 1997; *2*(6): 568–571.

Aluoch JR. The presence of sickle cells in the peripheral blood film. Specificity and sensitivity of diagnosis of homozygous sickle cell disease in Kenya. *Trop Geogr Med* 1995; *47*(2): 89–91.

AMA Council Report: Guidelines for handling parenteral anti-neoplastics. *JAMA* 1985; 233(11):1590–1592.

American Society of Hospital Pharmacists Technical Assistance Bulletin on Handling Cytotoxic and Hazardous Drugs. *Am J Hosp Pharm* 1990; 47:1033–1049.

Angelkort B, Maurin N, Booteng K. Influence of pentoxifylline on erythrocyte deformability in peripheral occlusive disease. *Curr Med Res Opin* 1979; 6:255–258.

Angelkort B. Thrombozytenfunktion, plasatische blutzerinnung und fibrinolyse bei chronisch aterieller verschluss kranheit. *Die Medizinische Welt* 1979; 30:1239–1243.

Armitage JO. Bone Marrow Transplantation. In: Fauci et al eds. *Harrison's Principles of Internal Medicine* 14th edition 1998. New York: McGraw-Hill: 724–730.

Assimadi JK, Gbadoe AD, Nyadanu M. The impact on families of sickle cell disease in Togo. *Arch Pediatr* 2000 Jun; 7(6): 615–620. (French)

Ataga KI, Orringer EP. Renal abnormalities in sickle cell disease. *Am J Hematol* 2000 Apr; 63(4):205–211.

Baird JK, Fryauff DJ, Basri H, Bangs MJ, Subianto B, Wiady I, Leksana B, Masbar S, Richie TL, Jones TR, Tjitra E, Wignall S, Hoffman SL. Primaquine for prophylaxis among nonimmune transmigrants in Irian Jaya, Indonesia. *Amer J Trop Med Hyg* 1995; 52(6): 479–484.

Ballas SK, Mohandas N. Pathophysiology of vaso-occlusion. *Hemat Oncol Clin North Am* 1996; 10:1221–1239.

Behrens RJ and Cymet TC. Sickle Cell Disorders: Evaluation, Treatment and Natural History. *Hospital Physician* 2000; 36:9.

Benjamin, G.C. Sickle Cell Anemia. *The Cambridge World History of Human Disease* 1993. Cambridge University Press.

Beutler E. Disorders of hemoglobin. In: Fauci et al eds. *Harrison's Principles of Internal Medicine* 14th edition 1998. New York: McGraw-Hill; 645–652.

Beutler E. The sickle cell diseases and related disorders. In: E

Beutler et al eds. *Williams Hematology*, 5th edition 1995. New York: McGraw-Hill; 616–654.

Bitanga E, Rouillon JD. Influence of sickle cell trait on energy and abilities. *Path Biol Paris* 1998 Jan; 46(1):46–52. Review (French).

Bloom, Miriam. *Understanding Sickle Cell Disease* 1999. Mississippi: University of Mississippi Press.

Boogaerts MA, Milbrain S, Meerus P, van Hove L, Verhoef GEG. In vitro modulation of normal human neutrophil function by pentoxifylline. *Blut* 1990; 61:60–65.

Bunn HF. Pathogenesis and treatment of sickle cell disease. *N Engl J Med* 1997; 337: 762–769.

Burlew K, Telfair J, Colangelo L, Wright EL. Factors that influence adolescent adaptation to sickle cell disease. *J Pediatr Psychol* 2000 Jul-Aug; 25(5):287–299.

Cao A. 1993 William Allan Award address. *Am J Hum Genet* 1994; 54:397–402.

Cartwright K. Meningococcal Carriage and Disease. In: 1995; K Cartwright ed. *Meningococcal Disease* 1995. K Cartwright ed. Chichester: John Wiley; 115–146.

Castro O, Brambilla DJ, Thorington B, et al. The acute chest syndrome in sickle cell disease: incidence and risk factors. The Cooperative Study of Sickle Cell Disease. *Blood* 1994; 84(2): 643–649.

Centers for Disease Control and Prevention: Health Information for International Travelers. *HHS publication no. (CDC)* 1996; 96–8280. Washington: US Department of Health and Human Services.

Cepeda ML, Allen FH, Cepeda NJ, Yang YM. Physical growth, sexual maturation, body image, and sickle cell disease. *J Natl Med Assoc* 2000 Jun; 92(1):10–14.

Chambers JB, Forsythe DA, Betrano SL, Iwinski HJ, Steflik DE. Retrospective review of osteoarticular in a pediatric sickle cell age group. *J Pediatr Orthop* 2000 Sept-Oct; 20(5):682–685.

Chang YP, Maier-Redelsperger M, Smith KD, et al. The relative importance of the X-linked FCP locus and beta-globin haplotypes in determining haemoglobin F levels: a study of SS patients homozygous for beta S haplotypes. *Br J Haematol* 1997; 96(4)L 806–814.

Chao NJ, Schmidt SM, Niland JC, Amylon MD, Dagis AC, Long GN, Nadananee AP, Negron RS, O'Donnell MR, Parker PM, Smith EP, Snyder DS, Stein AS, Wong RM, Blume KG, Forman SJ. Cyclosporine, methotrexate, and prednisone compared with cyclosporine and prednisone for prophylaxis of acute graft-vs-host disease. *N Engl J Med* 1993; 329.1225–1230.

Charache S, Barton FB, Moore RD, Terrin ML, Steinberg MH, Dover GJ, Ballas SK, McMahon RP, Castro O, Orringer EP. Hydroxyurea and sickle cell anemia. Clinical utility of a myelosuppressive "switching" agent. The Multicenter Study of Hydroxyurea in Sickle Cell Anemia. *Medicine* 1996; 75(6):300–326.

Charache S, Dover GJ, Moore RD, Eckert S, Ballas SK, Koshy M, Millner PF, Orringer EP, Phillips G Jr., Platt OS, Thomas GU. Hydroxyurea: Effects on hemoglobin F production in patients with sickle cell anemia. *Blood* 1992; 79:2555–2565.

Cipolotti R, Caskey MF. Childhood and adolescent growth of patients with sickle cell disease in Arlogs, Sergipe North East Brazil. *Ann Trop Pediatrics* 2000 June; 20(2):109–113.

Clark, Cathy. Gene Therapy A Promising New Strategy for Sickle Cell Anemia. *Blood Weekly* 1998; 13.

Clift RA, Bucker CD, Appelbaum FR, Schoch G, Peterson FB, Bensinger FB, Senders WJ, Sullivan RM, Storb R, Singer J. Allogeneic marrow transplantation during untreated first relapse of acute myeloid leukemia. *J Clin Oncol* 1992; 1723–1729.

Clinical Oncological Society of Australia: Guidelines and Recommendations for Safe Handling of Antineoplastic Agents. *Med J Australia* 1983; 1:426–428.

Consensus Conference. Newborn screening for sickle cell disease and other hemoglobinopathies. *JAMA* 1987; 258(9):1205–1209.

Controlling Occupational Exposure to Hazardous Drugs. (OSHA Work Practice Guidelines). *Am J Health-Syst Pharm* 1996; 53:1669–1685.

Crystal RG. Transfer of genes to humans. Early lessons and obstacles to success. *Science* 1995; 270:404–410.

Davies SM, Shu XO, Blazav AH, Filipovich JH, Kersey JH, Krivit W, McCullough J, Miller WJ, Ramsay NKC, Segall M, Wagner JE, Weisdorf DJ, McGlave PB. Unrelated donor bone marrow transplantation: Influence of HLA A and B incompatibility on outcome. *Blood* 1995; 86:1636–1642.

Davis H, Moore RM Jr, Gergen PJ. Cost of hospitalizations associated with sickle cell disease in the United States. *Public Health Rep* 1997; 112(1): 40–43.

Dormandy J, Nash GB, Loosemore T, Thomas PR. Effects of acute Trental on white cell rheology in patients with critical leg ischemia. In: J Hakim, GL Mandell, WJ Novick Jr eds. *Pentoxifylline and Analogues: Effects on Leukocyte Function* 1990. Basel, Switzerland: S. Karger; 203–205.

Egrie JC, Strickland TW, Lane J, Aoki K, Cohen AM, Smalling R, Trail G, Lin FK, Browne JK, Hines DK. Characterization and biological effects of recombinant human erythropoietin. *Immunobiol*,1986; 172:213–224.

Ehlers KH, Giardina PJ, Lesser ML, Engle MA, Hilgartner MW. Prolonged survival in patients with beta-thalassemia treated with deferoxamine. *J Pediatr* 1991; 118:540–545.

Embury SH et al eds. *Sickle Cell Diseases: Basic Principles and Clinical Practice* 1994. Hagerstown, MD: Lippincott-Raven.

Eschbach JW, Egrie JC, Downing MR, Brown JK, Adamson JW. The use of recombinant human erythropoietin (r-HuEPO). Effect in end-stage renal disease (ESRD). In Friedman, Boyer, DeSanto, Giordano eds. *Prevention of Chronic Uremia* 1989. Philadelphia, PA: Field and Wood Inc; 149–155.

Eschbach JW, Egrie JC, Downing MR, Browne JK, Adamson JW. Correction of the anemia of end-stage renal disease with recombinant human erythropoietin. *N Eng J Med* 1987; 316(2):73–78.

Fedson DS, Musher DM. Pneumococcal vaccine. In: SA Plotkin, EA Mortimer Jr eds. *Vaccines* 2nd edition 1994. Philadelphia: Saunders; 517.

Ferrari E, Fioravanti M, Patti AL, Viola C. Effects of long term treatment (four years) with pentoxifylline on hemorrheological changes and vascular complications in diabetic patients. *Pharmatherapeutica* 1987; 5:26–39.

Fleming DR, Rayens NK, Garrison J. Impact of obesity on allogeneic stem cell transplant patients: A matched case-controlled study. *Am J Med* 1997; 102(3):265–268.

Frasch CE. Meningococcal vaccines: Past, present, and future. In: K Cartwright ed. *Meningococcal Disease* 1995. Chichester: John Wiley; 35–70.

G.R. Serjeant. Sickle cell disease. *Lancet* 1997; 350: 725–730.

Gaston MH, Verter JL, Woods G, et al. Prophylaxis with oral penicillin in children with sickle cell anemia: a randomized trial. *N Engl J Med* 1986; 314:1593–1599.

Gill FM, Sleeper LA, Weiner SJ, et al. Clinical events in the first decade in a cohort of infants with sickle cell disease. The Cooperative Study of Sickle Cell Disease. *Blood* 1995; 86(2): 776–783.

Glickman E, Horowitz MM, Chanopin RE, Hows JM, Bacigalapo A, Biggs JL, Camitta BM, Gale RP, Gordon-Smith LC, Marmont AM, Masuoka T, Ramsay NKC, Rima A, Rozman C, Sabocinski KA, Speck B, Bortin MM. Bone marrow transplantation for severe aplastic anemia: Influence of conditioning and severe graft-vs-host disease prophylaxis regimens on outcome. *Blood* 1992; 79:269–275.

Goldstein M. *The Nature of Animal Healing* 1999. New York: Alfred A Knopf; 216–217.

Graber SE, Krantz SB. Erythropoietin and the control of red cell production. *Ann Rev Med* 1978; 29:51–58.

Grant MM, Gill KM, Floyd MY, Abrams M. Depression and functioning in relation to health care use in sickle cell disease. *Ann Behav Med* 2000 Spring; 22(2):149–157.

Gucalp R, Dutcher J. Oncologic Emergencies. In Fauci et al eds. *Harrison's Principles of Internal Medicine* 14th edition 1998. New York: McGraw-Hill; 627–634.

Hillman RS. Iron deficiency and other hypoproliferative anemias. In: Fauci et al eds. *Harrison's Principles of Internal Medicine* 14th edition 1998. New York: McGraw-Hill; 638–645.

Hiruma H, Noguchi CT, Uyesaka N, Hasegawa S, Blanchette-Mackie EJ, Schecter AN, Rodgers GP. Sickle cell rheology is determined by polymer fraction-not cell morphology. *Am J Hematol* 1995; 48(1):19–28.

Ibidapo MO, Akinyaju OO. Acute sickle cell syndromes in Nigerian adults. *Clin Lab Hematol* 2000 Jun; 22(3):151–155.

Israel RA, Rosenberg HM, Curtin LR. Analytical potential for multiple cause-of death data. *Am J Epidemiol* 1986; 124:161–79.

Itoh T, Chien S, Usami S. Effects of hemoglobin concentration on individual sickle cells after deoxygenation. *Blood* 1995; 85:2245–2253.

Jean-Baptiste GA, Leuleer K. Osteoarticular disorders of hematological origin. *Baillieres Best Pract Res Clin Rheumatol* 2000 Jun; 14(2):307–323.

Jim RTS. New therapy for microangiopathic hemolytic anemia caused by cardiac valve prosthesis: a case report. *Hawaii Med J* 1988; 47:285.

Jones RB, Frank R, Mass T. Safe handling of chemotherapeutic agents: a report from The Mount Sinai Medical Center. *CA Cancer J Clin* 1983; 33(5):258–263.

Kachmaryk MM, Trimble SN, Gieser RG. Cilioretinal artery occlusion in sickle cell trait. *Retina* 1995; 15:501–504.

Kark JA, Posey DM, Schumacher HR and Ruehle CJ. Sickle-cell trait as a risk factor for sudden death in physical training. *N Engl J Med* 1987; 317:781–786.

Krause PJ, Maderazo KG, Contrino J, Eisenfeld L, Herson VC, Greca N, Bannon P, Kreutzer DL. Modulation of neonatal neutrophil function by pentoxifylline. *Pediatr Res* 1991; 29:123–127.

Ladwig P, Murray H. Sickle cell disease in pregnancy. *Aust NZ J Obstet Gynecol* 2000 Feb; 40(1):97–100.

Leiken SL, Gallagher D, Kinney TR et al. Mortality in children and adolescents with sickle cell disease. The Cooperative Study of Sickle Cell Disease. *Pediatrics* 1989; 84(3): 500–508.

Lell B, May J, Schmidt RJ. The role of red blood cell polymorphism in resistance and susceptibility to malaria. *Ann Infect Dis* 1999 Apr; 28(4):794–799.

Leohardt H, Grigolet HG. Effects of pentoxifylline on red blood cell deformability and blood viscosity under hyperosmolar conditions. *Naunyn Schniedebergs Arch Pharmacol* 1977; 299:197–200.

Lorey F, Cunningham, Shafer F, Lubin B and Vichinsky E. Universal screening for hemoglobinopathies using high-performance liquid chromatography: clinical results of 2.2 million screens. *Eur J Hum Genet* 1994; 2:262–271.

Lorey FW, Arnopp J and Cunningham G. Distribution of hemoglobinopathy variants by ethnicity in a multiethnic state. *Genet Epidemiol* 1996; 13:501–512.

Lucarelli G, Galimberti M, Polchi P, Angelucci E, Barancianci D, Giardini C, Politi P, Durazzi SM, Muretto P, Albertini F. Bone marrow transplantation in patients with thalassemia. *N Engl J Med* 1990; 322:417–421.

Lundin AP, Akerman MJH, Chester RM. Exercise in hemodialysis patients after treatment with recombinant human erythropoietin. *Nephron* 1991; 58:315–319.

Marshall E. Gene therapy's growing pains. *Science* 1995; 269:1050–1055.

Mohan JS, Vigilance JE, Marshall JM, Hambleton IR, Reid HL, Serjeany GR. Abnormal venous function in patients with homozygous sickle cell (SS) disease and chronic leg ulcers. *Clin Sci* (Colch) 2000 Jun; 98(6):667–672.

Mortality among children with sickle cell disease identified by newborn screening during 1990–1994–California, Illinois and New York. *MMWR* 1998; 47(9): 169–172.

Muller R. Hemorheology and peripheral vascular disease: a new therapeutic approach. *J Med* 1981; 12:209–235.

Musher DM. Pneumococcal Infections. In: Fauci et al eds. *Harrison's Principles of Internal Medicine* 14th edition 1998. New York: McGraw-Hill; 869–875.

Nagel RL and Ranney HM. Genetic epidemiology of structural mutations of the beta-globin gene. *Semin Hematol* 1990; 27(4): 342–359.

National Institutes of Mental Health. *Recommendations for the Safe Handling of Parenteral Antineoplastic Drugs.* (NIH Publication No. 83–2621.) For sale by the Washington, DC: U.S. Government Printing Office

National Sickle Cell Anemia Control Act of 1972. Public Law 92–294, 86 Stat. 138.

National Study Commission on Cytotoxic Exposure. *Recommendations for Handling Cytotoxic Agents* (n.d.). Boston: Massachusetts College of Pharmacy and Allied Health Sciences.

Neonato MG, Guillod-Batalle M, Beauvais P, Beguei P, et al. Acute clinical events in 299 homozygous sickle cell patients living in France. French Study Group on Sickle Cell Disease. *Eur J Hematol* 2000 Sept; 65(3):155–164.

New York Newsday, Wednesday, Dec 1,1999:A38 (compiled from news dispatches).

Newborn Screening Committee, The Council of Regional

Networks for Genetic Services (CORN). National Newborn Screening Report-1993. Atlanta: CORN, 1998.

Nissenson AR, Nimer SD, Wolcott DL. Recombinant human erythropoietin and renal anemia:molecular biology, clinical efficacy and nervous system effects. *Ann Int Med* 1991; *114*(5):402–416.

Nwadiaro HC, Ugwu BT, Legbo JN. Chronic osteomyelitis in patients with sickle cell disease. *East Afr Med J* 2000 Jun; 77(1):23–26.

Ogandi SO, Onwe F. A pilot survey comparing the level of sickle cell disease knowledge in a university of South Texas and a university in Enugu, Enugu state, Nigeria, West Africa. *Ethn Dis* 2000 Spring-Summer; *10*(2):232–236.

Ohne-Frempong K, Weiner SJ, Sleeper LA, et al. Cerebrovascular accidents in sickle cell disease: Rates and risk factors. *Blood* 1998; *91*(1): 288–294.

Online Mendelian Inheritance in Man (OMIMTM). MIM Number: 141900: 6–26–98. Johns Hopkins University, Baltimore, MD. WWW URL: http://www.ncbi.nlm.nih.gov/omim/

Pathophysiology and management of sickle cell pain crisis. Report of a Meeting of Physicians and Scientists, University of Texas Health Science Center at Houston, Texas. *Lancet* 1995; 346:1408–1411.

Sifton et al. eds. *Physicians' Desk Reference* 53rd edition 1999. Montvale NJ: Medical Economics Inc; 774–775.

Platt OS, Brambilla DJ, Rosse WF, et al. Mortality in sickle cell disease- Life expectancy and risk factors for early death. *N Engl J Med* 1994; 330(23): 1639–1644.

Powars D and Hiti A. Sickle cell anemia. Beta s gene cluster haplotypes as genetic markers for severe disease expression. *Am J Dis Child* 1993; *147*(11): 1197–1202.

Fauci et al eds. *Principles of Internal Medicine*, 14th edition 1998. New York: McGraw-Hill; 910–915.

Rahimy MC, Gangboa A, Adjou R, Deguenon C, Goussanou S, Ahihonou E. Effect of active management on pregnancy outcome in sickle cell disease in an African setting. *Blood* 2000 Sept 1; 96(5):1685–1689.

Sacerdote A, Bishnoi A. Enhanced reduction of proteinuria in diabetics with triple therapy: pentoxifylline, protein restriction, and angiotensin converting enzyme inhibitors. *Diabetes* 1989; 38(supp):158A.

Sacerdote A, Bishnoi A. Triple therapy for proteinuria in diabetics; pentoxifylline, protein restriction, and angiotensin converting enzyme inhibitors. *Clin Res* 1989; 37:860A.

Sacerdote A, Rodriguez M. Treatment of homozygous SS disease with pentoxifylline. *Clin Res* 1994; 42:239A.

Sacerdote A. Treatment of homozygous sickle cell disease with pentoxifylline. *J Natl Med Assoc* 1999; 91(9):466–470.

Schnetterer L, Kemmler D, Breitenender H, Alschinger C, Koppensteiner R, Lexer F, Fercher AF, Eichler H, Wolgt M. A randomized, placebo-controlled, double-blind crossover of the effect of pentoxifylline on ocular fundus pulsations. *Am J Opthal* 1996; 121:169–176.

Schubolz R, Mufellner O. The effect of pentoxifylline on erythrocyte deformability and phosphatide fatty acid distribution in the erythrocyte membrane. *Curr Med Res Opin.* 1977; 4:609–617.

Segal, M. New Hope for Children with Sickle Cell Anemia Disease. *FDA Consumer* 1989 March.

Shanks GD. Malaria Prevention and Prophylaxis. In: G Pasvol ed. *Balliere's Clinical Infectious Diseases* vol. 2–2 1995. London: Balliere Tindall; 331–349.

Shapiro ED, Berg AT, Austrian R, Schroeder D, Parcells V, Margolis A, Adair RK, Clemens JD. The protective efficacy of polyvalent pneumococcal polysaccharide vaccine. *N Eng J Med* 1991; 325:1453–1460.

Sickle Cell Disease Guideline Panel. *Sickle cell disease: screen -*

ing, diagnosis, management, and counseling in newborns and infants. *Clinical Practice Guideline No. 6.* (AHCPR Pub. No. 93–0562.) Rockville, MD: Agency for Health Care Policy and Research, Public Health Service, U.S. Department of Health and Human Services. April 1993.

Silverstien, Alvin and Virginia. *Sickle Cell Anemia* 1997. Springfield, NJ: Enslow Publishers, Inc.

Simberkoff MS, Cross AP, Al-Ibrahim M, Baltch AL, Geiseler PJ, Nadler J, Richmond AS, Smith RP, Schiffman G, Shepard DS, Van Eeckhout JP. Efficacy of pneumococcal vaccine in high-risk patients. Results of a Veteran Administration Cooperative Study. *N Eng J Med* 1986; 315(21):1318–1327.

Snyder HW, Mittelman A, Oral A, Messerschmidt GL, Henry DH, Henry DH, Korec S, Bertran JH, Guthrie TH Jr, Ciarella D, Wurst D, Perkins W, Balint JP Jr, Cochran SK, Pengout R, Jones FR. Treatment of cancer chemotherapy-associated thrombotic thrombocytopenic/hemolytic uremic syndrome by protein A immunoadsorption of plasma. *Cancer* 1993; 71(5):1882–1892.

Solberg CO. Meningococcal Infections. In: Fauci et al eds. *Harrison's Principles of Internal Medicine* 14th edition 1998. New York: McGraw-Hill.

Solerte SB, Ferrari E. Diabetic retinal vascular complications and erythrocyte flexibility: results of a two year follow-up study with pentoxifylline. *Pharmatherapeutica* 1985; 4:341–349.

Steketee RW, Wirima JJ, Slutsker L, Khoromana CO, Heymann DL, Breman JG. Malaria treatment and prevention in pregnancy: The indications for use and adverse events associated with use of chloroquine and mefloquine. *Am J Trop Med Hyg* 1996; *suppl*: 50–56.

Thomas PW, Higgs DR and Serjeant GR. Benign clinical course in homozygous sickle cell disease: a search for predictors. *J Clin Epidemiol* 1997; 50(2): 121–126.

Treacy E, Childs B, Scriver CR. Response to treatment in hereditary metabolic disease. *Am J Hum Genet* 1995; 56(2):359–367.

Valle D. Treatment and Prevention of Genetic Disease. In: Fauci et al eds. *Harrison's Principles of Internal Medicine*, 14th edition 1998. New York: McGraw-Hill; 403–409.

Walters MC, Ohene-Frempong K, Patience M, Leisenring W, Eckman JR, Scott JP, Mentzer WC, Davies SC, Bernandin F, Matthews DC, Storb R, Sullivan KM. Bone marrow transplantation for sickle cell disease. *N Engl J Med* 1996; 335:369–376.

Walters MC, Patience M, Leisenring W, Rogers ZR, et al. Collaborative multicenter investigation of marrow transplantation for sickle cell disease: current results and future directions. *Biol Blood Marrow Transplant* 1997; 3(6): 310–315.

Wethers DL. Sickle cell disease in childhood. Part II. Diagnosis and treatment of major complications; recent advances in treatment. *Am Fam Phys* 2000 Sept 15; 62(6):1309–1314.

Wun T, Paglieroni T, Field CL, Welborn J, Cheung A,Walker NJ, Tablin F. Platelet-erythrocyte adhesion in sickle cell disease. *J Invest Med* 1999; 47(3):121–127.

Xu, K., Rosenwaks, Z. First Unaffected Pregnancy Using Preimplantation Genetic Diagnosis for Sickle Cell Anemia. *JAMA* 1999 May 12.

Yardley-Jones A. What are the implications of sickle cell anemia? *Occup Med* (London) 1999 Jan; 49(1): 55–56.

Zimmerman SA, Ware RE. Palpable splenomegaly in children with hemoglobin SC disease. Hematological and clinical manifestations. *Clin Lab Hematol* 2000 Jun; 22(3):145–156.

INDEX

children at risk for strokes and, 107

complications, 183–187

cost of, 78, 181

future of, 187–188

marrow graft rejection, 184

matching tissue types, 179–180

National Marrow Donor Program, 179–180

post-transplantation care, 182–183

preparing for, 182

qualifying for, 180–181

risks of, 178, 181

transplantation explained, 181–183

bone pain, 42, 149

bones

abnormal development of jaw and breast bone, 120

books, recommended, 217–221

BUN (blood urea nitrogen) test, 84

caffeine, 46

camps, summer, 119, 199

cancer, screening for, 150

capillaries, 7, 41

career choices, for teenagers, 145–146

carrier, 224

case studies (personal narratives)

adult with sickle cell disease, 147–149, 153–157

parents that carry sickle cell trait, 29–33

stem cell transplant, 177–178

taking charge of treatment, 195–196

teenager with sickle cell disease, 131–132

young adult with sickle cell disease, 139–141

CBC. *See* complete blood count

CD ROMs, 216–217

chaplains, 74

chelation therapy, for iron overload, 88–89

chest pain, and children, 109

children

ages birth–6 months old, 97–98

ages 6–12 years old, 98

common manifestations, 101–103

healthy diet, principles for, 60–62

talking about chronic disease with, 33–34, 99

teachers, guidelines for, 127–129

what to do when they act out, 100–101

chorionic villus sampling (medical test), 23

chromosome, 224–225

climate considerations, and sickle cell disease, 58